M.I.N.D.
OVER
WEIGHT®

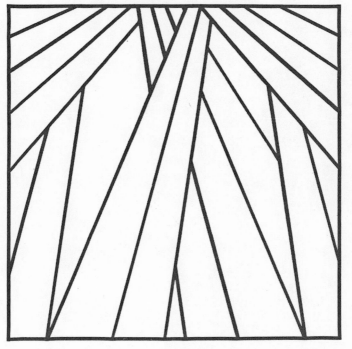

William M. Macleod
and Gael S. Macleod

M.I.N.D.
OVER
WEIGHT®

How to
Stay Slim
the Rest
of Your Life

PRENTICE-HALL, INC., Englewood Cliffs, New Jersey

10 9 8 7 6 5 4 3 2 1

Library of Congress Cataloging in Publication Data
Macleod, William M.   date
M.I.N.D. over weight®

1. Reducing–Psychological aspects.   2. Self-control.
3. Mind and body.   I.   Macleod, Gael S.,
date   joint author.   II.   Title.
RM222.2.M23   616.3'9805   80-21001
ISBN 0-13-583385-X

Contents

To our children,
Lorna, Gary, David, and Michael.

Preface

by Alfred Weiss, Ph.D., Associate Professor, City College of New York, Certified Psychologist

It's a fair assumption that people in this country lose millions of pounds every year. It's also fair to assume that most people gain back the pounds they lose. Since at least several books each year offer the "diet to end all diets," what, then, is so novel about another book aimed at the control of overweight?

The simple truth is that weight loss occurs when more calories are burned up than are ingested (except where certain physiological problems interfere seriously with the system and require medical attention). The age-old question has been, How does one control eating habits so that, indeed, fewer calories are eaten than are used up in activity?

Herein lies the novelty of the Macleods' approach. Their method is free of exhortation concerning drugs, use of special products, or adherence to rigid, possibly confining diets. Through the M.I.N.D. OVER WEIGHT® process, individuals are given pragmatic principles and techniques which enable them to con-

9

front their disabling lack of control and to reestablish a sense of self-respect and self-assertiveness with respect to their bodies. These techniques are derived from the Macleods' many years of practice and teaching.

You will note a repetition of the word *self* in the previous paragraph. That is because the Macleods have based their method on an intrinsic respect for the determination of each individual to establish control over his or her own life, as well as his or her own eating habits. For them, this determination is not created through rigid adherence to faddist diets; rather, it develops naturally through a process of self-awareness and self-affirmation. In placing the locus of control in the individual rather than the diet, the Macleods deal frankly and informatively with the basic anxieties and conflicts that obstruct permanent weight loss. And in doing so, they encourage the individual's determination to both lose weight and maintain the loss.

There will never be a simple "tomorrow-you-will-be-completely-cured" road to self-knowledge and change. However, by emphasizing the positive experience of becoming a more complete person and of utilizing the self effectively, the M.I.N.D. OVER WEIGHT® method encourages self-determination not only in the area of weight control, but in many other aspects of life as well.

In that regard, successful use of M.I.N.D. OVER WEIGHT® can prove to be one of the few experiences in life in which a permanent loss is also a very personal gain.

I heartily recommend it to you.

Foreword

by Lester W. Eisenstodt, M.A. (Ed.), M.A.,
M.D., F.I.C.S., F.A.C.S., F.A.A.F.P.R.S.,
D.I.B.S., D.A.B., Senior Attending,
Department of General Surgery,
Division of Plastic Surgery,
St. Michael Medical Center

M.I.N.D. OVER WEIGHT® is a bright new book which teaches one to control the mind to program the amount of food ingested each day. The method is one of constructive relaxation, which simultaneously coordinates the mind, the mirror, the body, and the scale. Through this process, the need for appetite-diminishing pills, strict dietary controls, and vigorous exercise is virtually eliminated. The psyche automatically stimulates one to eat sensibly and assesses the quantity and quality of food to be consumed in order to obtain and then *maintain* the desired body weight.

The method works. I have personally witnessed the successful use of its techniques, as my wife was one of William Macleod's students. Prior to his teaching, she was a yo-yo gal who lost and regained too many pounds to mention. By practicing his M.I.N.D. OVER WEIGHT® method, she learned how to automatically coordinate her mind and body to ingest the amount of food necessary for her to first lose and then maintain her desired body contour. In her own words, she is now "slim, trim, and happy .. doing just beautifully."

As a plastic surgeon, coming in contact with many people desirous of improving their outer appearance, I am intimate with the problems that beset the overweight person. The Macleods' approach has been effective in weight control because it teaches one to solve his or her problem from within.

When an individual learns to control his or her mind, everything else becomes spontaneous. One achieves permanent weight loss by self-inculcating the desire to stay thin. Self-assessment, self-determination, and finally, self-indoctrination comprise the Macleods' prescribed method for using the mind to overcome one's weight problem.

Reflection, desire, and practical application are my Rx for its success.

Introduction

It was in the winter of 1971 when I first met Gael, and I was attracted to her instantly. There was something about her that was so refreshing. She was a warm and charming twenty-six-year-old woman with boundless energy. She was witty... always smiling... so eager to do nice things for other people. Her zest for life seemed real, and she appeared to be happy.

But as I got to know her better, I realized that the witty remarks, the constant smile, the attempts to please everybody were disguising her real feelings. She gave the appearance of a smiling, confident, and happy person, but underneath the surface lay other emotions—worry, fear, and a feeling of helplessness about her overweight condition.

At that time Gael weighed almost two hundred pounds, and she was going through the agonies of trying to lose some of them. She was beginning another diet. Moreover, I discovered that this was not new to her. It was an old, familiar pattern—a drama she had acted out many times before; so many times, in fact, that she had begun to live the part she was playing.

Beneath the happy exterior, I sensed a very frightened woman who spent most of her waking hours constantly struggling with a weight problem, fighting the clichéd battle of the bulge, and losing the war. This was her sixteenth year of being overweight, and nearly her hundredth attempt to keep it off. Yet deep down she knew before she got started on a new diet that it wasn't going to work. She'd acted the part enough to know what the end of the play would be— she'd gain back every pound she had fought hard to lose.

Nonetheless, she'd start a new restricting diet, and soon she would get anxious about being able to stick to it. If her resolve weakened and she broke the diet, it would send her to the refrigerator or on a frantic drive to the supermarket as if directed by some unseen force.

Whenever Gael got to the point where she couldn't stop eating, she'd look to her overweight friends for support—people who understood because they'd been there themselves, or who were sympathetic listeners. And there were the endless trips to her local weight-loss center too, where she'd be complimented on her progress or consoled upon the slightest setback. But whatever happened really didn't matter since Gael was a compulsive eater, and she'd always wind up celebrating her successes—or feeding her failures—by picking up a pizza or an ice-cream cake, or whatever else she had been forbidden under the rules of whichever weight-loss program she was exploring.

Eventually this compulsive eating would catch

up with her. She would step on the scale or look at herself in the mirror and come face to face with her moment of truth. It was happening again—she was gaining back the weight! She'd throw up her arms in desperation, saying, "I've been overweight all my life . I'll never be thin."

So she'd give up her diet—again.

Assuming the role of being overweight, she was certain she would be fat and unhappy for the rest of her life. It was almost impossible for her to imagine herself thin. Besides, playing the overweight role was easy. She was more than just comfortable in it—she was a *star!*

It was a part, though, that didn't make her happy. A simple invitation to go out to dinner with friends would throw her into a frenzy. Trying to find an outfit to wear that would hide her body was nearly impossible. Looking at herself in the mirror while dressing for dinner became a nightmare, and trying to nibble tiny portions of food while everybody at the dinner table ate to their heart's content became an agony.

Soon she resisted going out at all, preferring to stay home. It became her prison, one filled with self-doubt, fear, and unhappiness. Her entire social life was collapsing as Gael, tormented by feelings of inadequacy and lack of control, locked herself deeper and deeper into a self-created solitary confinement.

What she really wanted to be was thin. That was the goal she set out to achieve every time she tried a new way to control her weight. And she had tried them all! Yet every time she looked at herself in the mirror, she saw herself as a failure, and it was affecting her entire life.

I ached for Gael as I saw her go through all of

this, and found myself wondering if she really knew what she was doing to herself. This was her life, and I wanted her to be happy in it.

I believed that all of life was meant to be enjoyed to the fullest. In order to achieve that, an individual must first like oneself. Clearly, Gael didn't like herself at all as I liked her. And as I saw the warm and wonderful woman she was, I found myself falling in love with her. She was a beautiful person, and it didn't matter to me that her body was in an overweight condition. However, it mattered to her; it mattered a lot. Surely, I thought, there had to be a permanent solution somewhere?

For the previous few years, I had been doing some work on myself. I described it as self-work in reference to the mind—my mind. I had been going through a difficult time, until one day it became apparent to me that certain of my inner attitudes and beliefs were causing my difficulties. I discovered they were holding me back from success. Indeed, they alone were deterring me in my pursuit of a healthy, happy life. I recognized them as my beliefs—a part of me. I had lived with them for many years, but I decided I could live with them no longer.

Thus I went about altering them by learning to use more of my mind than I had imagined possible before. The results were incredible! The circumstances hadn't changed, but my *perception* of them—and myself *in* them—became clearer. Thereafter, I found I could deal with my problems more effectively. Life no longer controlled me; I controlled my life. The self-work method proved its worth to me—it gave me a greater awareness of life and my role in it; it helped me to achieve one of my own lifetime goals. I reasoned it might help Gael in her pursuit of becoming and staying thin forever.

So I wondered: Could I teach Gael to use more of her mind in this way? Could these techniques of mind convince her that she was capable of becoming a thin person—without history repeating itself, without restricting diets, and without the fear of gaining back the weight?

M.I.N.D. OVER WEIGHT® was created for Gael, and it proved to be her salvation. Within ten months, Gael had trimmed down to a perfect 125-pound, happy, healthy woman who was no longer a compulsive eater. Now, almost nine years later, Gael has maintained her weight loss. What's more, she has found her lasting success without the frustration and agonizing restrictions of a weight-loss regimen, or diet. Gael, who is now my slim wife, can eat whatever she desires, whenever she desires, without the fear of becoming overweight.

Gael and I have been teaching the method to other overweight people for years, and we've had the privilege of seeing them attain a newfound freedom from fat—quickly, naturally, and permanently. We've written this book to bring these techniques to the many others who can benefit from its lessons.

M.I.N.D. OVER WEIGHT® can help you, too, just as it's helped hundreds we've known who were trapped in the overweight struggle.

William M. Macleod

Acknowledgments

To dear Al Weiss, whose wisdom and guidance, strong, loving support, and sense of humor saw us through it all.

And:

To "Mum," a mother who never let the distance become a gap, and who has always brought good fortune to our life.

To Papa and Florence, thanks for being such good parents.

To Elaine Kempen and Archie Macleod, whose love we never forget.

To "Bobonne," our dear grandmother, with love.

To Gerald Kempen and Donald Macleod, our brothers, who always had faith.

To Michael Ploshnick, always a friend.

To Taruna, for her sweet support and help when it was needed.

To Lou and Nancy Mercurio, for their enduring friendship.
To Fran Heller Glantz, for her assistance in organizing the book.
To Lee, and his zest for life.
To Dale Rappaport, for her kind advice at those opportune times.
To William T. Low, David Goldin, and Bill Zanowitz—endless thanks.
Special gratitude to Saul Cohen, our editor, who encouraged us to write this book.
We will never forget all our students over the years, who taught us so much.

To Life.

Chapter 1
DIETS ONLY LAST FOREVER

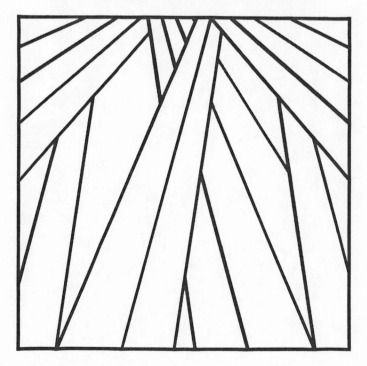

I know what you've been going through, and you know the routine by heart.

Think about it...

You're overweight. Whether it's five or fifty pounds, it doesn't really matter how much. You want to lose them. So you go on a diet. You lose a couple of pounds. In fact, you even may be successful and reach your ultimate goal—that magic number on the scale that informs you, "You've finally done it! Congratulations! It's time to celebrate."

Then you go off your diet, right back to the same old eating habits that made you overweight in the first place. Do you remember all the weight you lost? Somehow it finds you again. Doesn't it?

Eventually, you try another diet, determined this time to stick to it. Perhaps you lose some weight; perhaps you don't. But sooner or later, you "go off" the diet, gaining back all the weight you struggled so hard to lose... and then some!

Up and down. Up and down. Like an elevator, a seesaw, a yo-yo.

When you stop to think about it, how many pounds—in total—have you gained and lost over the years with some form of dieting? You probably don't know... it would be too depressing.

That's the diet syndrome, sampling one diet after another. The list of them is long: high protein, low carbohydrate, low fat, no fat, diet pills, diet aids, diet clubs, doctors' quick diets, crash diets. It's enough to make you want to raid the refrigerator, which you usually do because you've done it all before, many times.

Remember the last diet you tried? That nicely laid out meal plan designed to help you lose weight? Of course you remember—the one where you had to eat the same bland, dull breakfast, lunch, and dinner every day of the week. It was boring, but it was working—you *were* losing weight. Then one night... it happened.

You had your evening meal—those carefully measured four ounces of poultry or fish. One slice of dry whole wheat bread. Half a cup of plain steamed vegetables (only the green, leafy ones, of course!). Tossed salad with one measly teaspoon of awful-tasting low-calorie dressing. All of it washed down by a diet soda that reminded you of medicine.

Anyhow, it was midnight. You were wide awake ...and you were *starving*. You watched TV restlessly, while your spouse slept on the couch. Being on a diet, you couldn't run to the kitchen for a snack during the commercials, even though you'd been so good. You didn't nibble, you didn't munch. Noshing was out. You'd sat there like a good soldier, in quiet desperation—*thinking* about food, dreaming about all the goodies you weren't allowed to eat, suffering because you weren't eating them, but they were on the TV!

A sideways glance assured you that your spouse was sound asleep. Confident that no one else was looking, you tiptoed to the kitchen and opened the squealing refrigerator door. You stood there and stared, smacking your lips. Finally you said to yourself, "Oh, what the hell!" You gave up, gave in, and stuffed your face.

Of course you're going to eat! It happens all the time. In fact, sometimes you even don't wait for the food to defrost. There is nothing as delectably chewy as frozen cake.

You became a midnight raider, a thief in the night. Of course, the only person you've really robbed was yourself. It didn't make you feel too good, but you kept on eating anyway.

Think about it...

Being a midnight raider is just part of the ups and downs of the diet syndrome. It's the beginning. You're on your way back up.

Sneak eating is your next step. It's a more sophisticated sort of cheating than midnight raids. In public, you diet...as long as you have an audience. You're the kind of dieter who sits in an Italian restaurant and orders a salad instead of spaghetti. You wouldn't dream of touching the garlic bread. You pick at your entrée like a bird—boneless breast of chicken *without* the parmigiana. When everyone else at the table orders cheesecake for dessert, you politely decline.

At home, later that night, when no one's watching, you pad into the kitchen and single-handedly *kill* a gallon of chocolate ice cream.

When you sneak-eat, you volunteer to go food shopping a lot, too. Your intent, of course, is just to pick up a few groceries, but you end up bringing home bagfuls of forbidden fruit. Strolling up and down the aisles, you polish off a box of cookies *before* you get to the checkout counter, paying the cashier for the empty carton!

If you're lucky, when you come home from the market, no one is there. Time to unpack. It's just you and a few of your favorite snacks you couldn't resist dropping into the shopping cart. So you grab them and run around the house, surreptitiously stashing the stuff into your secret hiding places, where no one will think of looking for food. Whether it's popcorn in the attic, potato chips in the garage or candy bars under the bed, you'll get to it eventually. Unless, of course, you forget the whereabouts of the stashes.

If you're unlucky, you get caught red-handed with the goodies. "It's for the kids, dear," you sing out when your spouse sees you unloading the Mallomars from the shopping bag. The next day, when your spouse is hungry for cookies and a glass of milk, there's not a single Mallomar left. "The kids ate them."

Sure they did.

Who are you kidding? Not the kids, and certainly not your spouse.

Think about it...

Once your sneak-eating becomes routine, overweight sets in again. Are you surprised? That's why chronic sneak-eaters usually wind up running into each other every week at the local diet-club meeting.

You've probably been to at least one....

The first thing you face is the giant weigh-in, but you've prepared for it. Everyone has. You skipped eating dinner that evening. In fact, you starved yourself all day to make up for the cheating you did during the week. You dressed deliberately for the occasion, too, in lightweight clothes—the lighter, the better, even if it is below freezing outside. At the meeting, you wait with other hopefuls for your turn. When you're next to first in line, you remove your shoes and belt. You strip off your jewelry and empty your pockets. After all, that loose change could add up to an extra half ounce.

Down to bare essentials, you gingerly step up on the scale. As you chitchat with the instructor, you nonchalantly shift your weight to one foot while she's not looking, hoping the scale registers two pounds less. Once your weight's recorded, you take your seat, careful to avoid sitting near anyone thinner than you. Momentarily, the instructor announces, "Our group has lost twenty-five pounds this week!"

Everyone cheers. You do, too, as long as you've been fortunate enough to have contributed, even slightly, to the twenty-five–pound loss. If, on the other hand, you gained a quarter of a pound, you get depressed. Sometimes you become depressed enough to drive over to the local late-night eatery after the meeting to drown your sorrows in a hot fudge sundae.

Usually when you walk into the restaurant, you see many familiar faces. Then you remember where you saw them before—at the diet-club meeting!

Of course it was hard staying on the diet for the week. It was the one subject occupying you morning, noon, and night for the seven previous days. What you could eat—that was boring. What you couldn't eat— *that was frustrating!* What a way to live! You couldn't even enjoy eating a meal with your family. Sunday breakfast? There they were, feasting on pancakes oozing with melted butter and maple syrup, while you were stuck with a poached egg on toast, feeling very much like an outsider. Then, to make matters worse, you were the one who ended up clearing the table of *their* sticky messes.

The rest of the day loomed before you. You couldn't look forward to lunch. You couldn't look forward to dinner. There was nothing you could eat on the diet that you really liked. Your taste buds screamed for satisfaction!

What could you do? Suffer through another day hungry and deprived, or give in, regretting it the next morning when you stepped on the scale?

To eat or not to eat isn't all there is to it. The diet syndrome also dictates what you can and cannot wear.

Think about it...

Take a look at your clothes closet. Do you have four different wardrobes? After you've played the diet game long enough, your wardrobe doesn't change with the seasons—it goes from "thin" to "just right" to "overweight" to "obscene."

You never seem to have enough closet space. You can't throw things out because you never know when you're going to have to wear that size again. You hate to go shopping for new clothes. You dread the very thought, but there are times you simply can't avoid it. When you go, you usually shop alone.

You don't want anyone with you when you're trying on clothes. You don't want anyone else's opinion. You don't want anyone's advice. In fact, you don't want help from anyone at all. Certainly not from that skinny salesgirl. She looks as if she never had a weight problem in her life.

To add to your frustration, there's not much of a selection from which to choose—not in *your* size, anyway. Even the dressing rooms seem too tight.

Finally, when you do manage to try on a couple of outfits, nothing fits well. You've narrowed the field of choices to two; neither of which makes you happy. Either you have to buy a dumpy-looking outfit that fits, but makes you *feel* dumpy, or you opt for something a bit more stylish that is one size small in the vain hope that you'll fit into it next week. After all, you *are* on a strict diet.

However, you wisely settle for the bigger outfit, instead of the better style. It covers your bulges, and at least, it fits. It's usually dark, too, because dark colors make you look thinner. It becomes your uniform, and you wear it everywhere you go.

Before you change into your street clothes, you take a long, last look at yourself in the dressing-room mirror, and you don't like what you see. Gritting your teeth, you swear to yourself that you're never going to let yourself get fat like this again. You vow that *this* time you're going to stick to your diet; *this* time you're going to lose the weight and you're going to *keep it off*. You'll start the diet next Monday.

But you know, Monday never comes.

Think about it...

How do you feel when you're on a diet? What's your life like? Are you happy?

You know how anxious you are. Aside from everything else you have to concern yourself with, you've got to worry about how much weight you have to lose, whether or not you'll be able to lose it, and (if you do lose it) whether or not you can keep it off! After all, you've never been able to do it before.

Yet, by its very nature, *this* diet—or any other diet regimen for that matter—is going to restrict you. It tells you what to eat, what not to eat, how much to eat, even *when* to eat. Ironically, all you ever *do* think about is food. Your diet becomes the central topic pervading your thoughts and conversations. You become *obsessed* with it, planning your life around it. And when you stop to think about it, being on it is a constant reminder that you're an overweight person, that you're different from everybody else. That you're not like "normal" people. Other people seem to be able to eat whatever they want, whenever they want to eat it, and never gain an ounce.

You're irritable all the time, too. Who wouldn't be? You're constantly depriving yourself of something you really want. The harder you try to keep up the constant vigil, obeying all the rules and regulations of your diet's restrictive regimen, the greater the internal pressure to break it, until it reaches a peak when you just can't take it anymore. What do you do? You indulge yourself. You eat. Eating is the most effective release you have from all of the tension. The diet syndrome has begun and you are doomed, it seems, to be forever fat.

It's a vicious cycle, this diet syndrome. It feeds on itself, reinforcing your feelings of failure and self-defeat. Every time you fail at a diet you begin the cycle anew; you're more convinced than before that you're always going to be overweight.

It is either that or you're going to have to diet *forever!* You're wise enough to know that you can't live your life on a diet, because you always end up losing the game, *not* the weight.

It's feast or famine: You're eating compulsively or starving to death. You're miserable when you're dieting and you're miserable when you're not. You're sick and tired of going up and down, up and down...like an elevator...a seesaw...a yo-yo.

There is another way, a way to lose weight and keep it off. You'll be able to do it. It's not difficult, but you must venture beyond the diet syndrome.

Chapter 2
BEYOND THE DIET SYNDROME

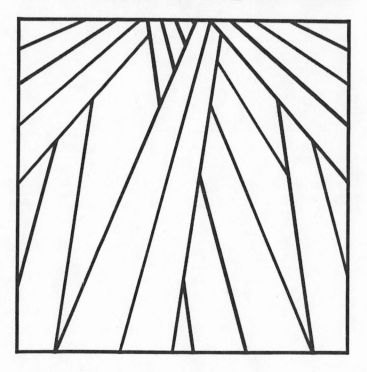

Beyond the realm of the diet syndrome is a wonderful place where you're free to live a happy life...a thin life. It's a place where you're in control, where you can eat whenever you want, whatever you want, and as much as you want, without fear of breaking a diet. It is a place where you won't be on a diet, and you will live without the fear of gaining weight.

Sound impossible? It's not. You just *believe* it is.

Think about it...

When you're trapped in the diet syndrome, it's very hard to envision what your life will be like beyond it. You don't believe you'll ever be able to get there.

Believe it. You can do it.

You'll be happier. Calmer. Free of worry. At peace with yourself. And you'll like yourself more.

You will be a thin person. Because being a thin person is what you really wanted to be all along. Otherwise, why would you have gotten yourself caught up in the diet syndrome? Until now, you never knew there was another way to lose weight, except for some form of dieting. Clearly, a diet can help you lose weight, but that's *all* it does. The secret is *keeping it off*...staying thin over the long haul. For years. Not months or weeks. That's what you've never been able to do. It doesn't mean you'll never be able to do it.

You have it within you to be thin and stay thin... forever. Somewhere deep down inside of you is a thin person who's desperately trying to get out. Find that person and you'll have the key that unlocks the door to the happy, thin life that lies beyond the diet syndrome. The way to get to that inner, thinner you is through a better understanding of yourself.

But before you can begin to understand how it can work for you—how you'll be able to use the M.I.N.D. OVER WEIGHT® method to get thin and stay thin forever—you first have to understand that your body is a reflection of your own unique self-image, that is, your concept of yourself. It mirrors in a real way your ideas about what you are and who you are as a person.

Just as you have opinions about other people, you have your own opinion about yourself. Think of your self-image as being your opinion of yourself. You may not be consciously aware of it, but it's *there* nonetheless. This image is constantly with you, like a photograph you carry around in your pocket. It's the mental blueprint for your entire life-style, mapped out in your mind. You behave according to it. You feel things because of it. It determines how you look, how you act, how you see your life, and your ability to make a success of it. All of your thoughts, emotions, and attitudes are a result of your self-image. It's what makes you *you*.

What is *your* self-image? What do you see when you look at yourself in the mirror? Take a moment, now, to do just that. It's important to your understanding of M.I.N.D. OVER WEIGHT®. Put the book down and study yourself in the mirror. Think objectively about the image reflected there; then come back.

What did you see?

Was there a happy, confident, and successful-looking person smiling at you from the glass? Did you notice all the nice things there were about that person? *How* did you see yourself?

The answer to this question defines your self-image, because the way you judge the person in the mirror is the way you see yourself. Also, the way you *feel* about the person in the mirror is the way you feel about yourself.

Self-image is not merely a surface concept. It is deeply embedded in your mind; it is an image that didn't develop overnight. It took its shape from all the beliefs you have about yourself, beliefs that took root and grew during your earliest years, when you weren't aware that they had been planted in your mind. Many of these beliefs came from people who were closest to you—your family, your friends, your teachers in school. Eventually, all of these beliefs became your own. Now they're yours, regardless of how they originated. Your self-image is the sum total of all these beliefs. It's what you truly believe yourself to be. Is it an unhappy, overweight person? A failure? Is that what you saw when you looked at yourself in the mirror?

Think about it...

Each time you diet and fail, what you're really doing is reinforcing the idea that you will never be thin, that you will always have a weight problem. In effect, you've programmed yourself to believe you will fail. Your deep inner belief that you'll always have a weight problem dictates failure in a vicious, circular pattern. You cannot hope to succeed if your self-image calls for failure, because buried deep in your mind is the belief that you are destined *not to win*.

Actually, self-image is a blueprint, no different than an architect's blueprint for a building. Without being aware of it, you design your own body in your mind, just as an architect designs a building on paper.

If the architect makes a mistake in the blueprint, the building will be erected with the same mistake repeated. If the architect catches the error before construction begins, then he can go back to the blueprint, correct the mistake, and confidently order the builder to proceed.

In the same way the builder can only build according to what his blueprint calls for, so your body can only reflect what your self-image is. If in your own mind you picture yourself as an overweight person, you will develop that picture in the form of an overweight body. Your mind will direct you to fulfill the image of "someone with a weight problem." Ultimately, it means you'll do whatever is necessary to achieve that self-image. You will overeat.

The singular reward for best performer in this kind of psychodrama is an extra roll of fat around the middle. As this overweight self-image solidifies in your mind, it solidifies on your body. Should you blame your body for this condition? Your body is simply obeying directions given it by your mind, based on the beliefs programmed into it. You'll never get beyond the diet syndrome this way.

Since you are the architect for your body through your mind, the concepts of M.I.N.D. OVER WEIGHT® will teach you how to use your mind to correct mistakes in your mental "blueprint," redesigning your faulty self-image, which your body will reflect.However, it is not enough to think positively to effect changes in your body. It isn't enough to endlessly repeat "I'm a thin person," when deep down your belief is really "I'll never be thin." That's like planting tulip bulbs in the fall, then expecting roses in the spring. It won't work. Your beliefs must be totally in unison with your thoughts. Changing your thoughts without changing your beliefs is merely working on the surface of the problem. Simply stated, you are what you *believe* you are, not what you think you are. There's a vast difference between thinking and believing.

•

Assume for a moment you want to repair a crack in your living-room wall. To save time and effort, you decide to paint it over. It works for a while because you no longer see the crack, but it will reappear eventually because the paint had nothing on which to adhere, the repair having been made only on the surface of the wall. However, if you had taken the time to sand down the wall and fill in the crack with compound before painting, you would have fixed the fissure permanently.

So it is with self-image. You not only have to think slim, but you have to believe it. Positive thinking works only on the surface problem; it doesn't remove permanently the faulty belief which lies beneath.

How many times in the past have you made a conscious decision to stop eating candy because you wanted to be thin, yet candy continued to be your downfall? "I *can* give it up," you assure yourself. "I've got will power. I can do it!" So you go to the movies, sauntering past the candy counter without so much as a second glance. You mean business. But as you sit inside the theater and watch the film, you find it increasingly difficult to ignore the sounds of the candy wrappers being torn open around you. Sooner or later that old feeling wells up inside you—the one that says,

"Movies aren't fun without candy!" The next thing you know, you're munching away on a huge chunk of chocolate. So much for positive thinking.

By the same token, it also doesn't work when you've made a conscious decision to eat "just one" of anything. "Just one" slice of pizza? Three slices later, you're wondering what in the world happened to your resolute will power?

Why didn't it work? Somewhere deep down, you didn't *believe* you would be able to control yourself. When you resolved to eat "just one," or none at all, you merely changed your thoughts, but you did not change your *beliefs*. Again, it's not enough to *think* that you can do it; you have to *believe* you can. Clearly, it's impossible to accomplish a positive thought when there's this voice somewhere inside constantly reminding you, "No. You can't. You always fail."

When your self-image is that of an overweight person, there is a constant struggle between your conscious attempts to think positively about getting thin and your deep-rooted beliefs which remind you that you cannot. In sum, your beliefs will win over your thoughts every time!

Your beliefs are so strong because they are like the roots of a tree... roots that give life to the tree. They determine the fullness of its branches, its beauty, and its health. Think about a healthy tree, full of foliage. See it in your mind. Then, suppose you notice it has one dead limb. There seems to be no apparent reason for its being there. After all, why would an otherwise healthy-looking tree have a single dead limb?

If you dug up the earth around the tree to find the root that corresponded to the dead branch and followed it to its end, you'd probably discover a mass of rock blocking the root from nourishment. The lesson is simple, really. When you look at a tree, you see only part of it: the trunk, the leaves, and the branches. The surface level. You don't see the roots because they go deeper.

It's the same with the roots of the beliefs in your mind; you're not consciously aware of them, either. Not all of them, anyway, but they're there, functioning continuously. Remember, your deep inner beliefs are controlling you—how you live, how you feel, how you look, how you behave, how your body functions, and how you eat. Every day of your life, every minute of the day—and just like the roots that control the health of the tree—your beliefs control your own self-image and consequent well-being. Block a root from growing, and the tree will produce a dead limb. Believe you're an overweight person, and your mind will produce an overweight body.

Your beliefs are that powerful. That deep-rooted. That much in control at all times. However, in the last analysis, they're only as strong as your desire to change them. You have the ability to change your beliefs whenever you want to, just as you have the ability to dig into the earth surrounding the tree in our analogy to find the blocked root that caused the dead limb. Similarly, you have the ability to dig deeper into your mind—deeper than you ever thought you could— to find the faulty belief that's causing your overweight self-image. If you remove the faulty belief that you'll always be an overweight person—freeing you to believe that you really can be thin—you'll begin to nourish your body differently. You'll adopt a healthier attitude toward food. You'll stop eating compulsively.

You'll start to feel better and look better. You'll be in control of your mind, your body, and your weight.

•

M.I.N.D. OVER WEIGHT® is the method that can help you change your faulty beliefs, by enabling you to discover the roots of your overweight problem. Like the tree, the mind operates on at least two levels: a surface—or conscious—level, and below the surface, at a subconscious level. It's in the subconscious where you'll find the roots of your own self-image and beliefs.

The subconscious plays an important role in your daily life. Unlike the conscious mind, it's with you constantly; it never sleeps. In sleep, your conscious mind's at rest while your subconscious remains hard at work. It assumes complete control, turning your thoughts into dreams, protecting your sleep. But when the alarm goes off, awakening you, your conscious mind springs into action. Even then, your subconscious does not now fall into sleep! It remains with you throughout the day. In fact, there are a lot of things you do without being aware you're doing them.

Suppose you pick up a cup of coffee poured five minutes ago, figuring the coffee has cooled down, but the cup's empty! What in the world happened to the coffee? Obviously, you drank it. You don't remember, because you were so engrossed in balancing your monthly checking-account statement, that you weren't consciously aware of picking up the coffee, let alone having drunk it. How many times have you done this with a coffee cake, instead of a coffee cup?

Many of the actions you call automatic are actually subconsciously produced. For example, when your head itches, you scratch it. Did you ever wonder how your hand happens to know exactly what it's supposed to do and where it's supposed to go? What tells it to reach up and scratch your head until the itch is gone? You do! Not consciously, of course. What it requires is the desire to get rid of the itch and the knowledge that scratching will do the job. Nothing more. It's your subconscious mind that carries out the desire and directs your hand. There is no complicated conscious process operating here; it's a simple subconscious process which carries out your commands. After all, you don't consciously tell yourself, "Oh, dear, I have an itch. I would like it to go away. So I will move my hand up to my head and move my fingers around until the itch is gone."

Your subconscious mind operates most of the time without your conscious awareness. You've probably experienced a subconscious level of awareness while driving a car. You're riding down the highway, not concentrating on driving the vehicle at all, just doing it. Your mind is occupied with other things: the problems you have with your boss or the kids, the weekend party that's coming up, your best friend's latest romance, that wonderful movie you saw. Or maybe you're reliving a past vacation: being back on that sunny beach...remembering the good time you had...relaxed...when your eye catches the exit sign and you realize you'd better move over or you'll miss your turnoff. You instantly snap back to reality. It's only then you realize you've been daydreaming for miles!

Whatever material you had in your subconscious had filtered into your conscious awareness while you were driving. It didn't interfere with your ability to operate the car. In fact, you were doing fine and you noticed the exit sign. Your mind was functioning well on two levels simultaneously. This is a perfect example of how different levels of the mind can operate in unison without your conscious awareness.

It is when the two levels go off in opposite directions that you run into trouble. That's precisely what happens when you are struggling to stay on a diet. The conscious and subconscious levels of your mind are not working in harmony. Your lips are singing, "No, no—don't eat," but there's "Yes, yes" on your mind.

Remember: *In order to be thin, you not only have to think, but you have to believe thin.* Since beliefs are rooted in the subconscious level, that's the place where permanent change can happen. If you consciously want to be thin and stay thin, you must change your subconscious, faulty belief that you'll always be overweight. It's the only way you'll be able to program pounds away quickly, naturally, and permanently, without ever consciously having to be on a diet.

Think about it...

Your mind acts like a computer. Consciously, you are the computer programmer, given all of this data: other people's thoughts, opinions, impressions, and beliefs, as well as your own. You feed this data into your mind to be sorted out, sometimes analyzed, and then stored in your subconscious, where it becomes a belief.

Recognize now that your mind has been *programmed*, by yourself and others, to believe you're an overweight person. The programming began at an early age. Perhaps you were a big baby. You heard your mother talking about how big you were when you were born, what a good eater you were, how you gained weight so fast. Even though you didn't understand what was happening, and had no defense against it, you took it all in, storing it away for future reference. As you grew older, you began to think of yourself as being big without being aware why.

When you were young, you didn't have much choice what went into your subconscious data bank. Your mind acted like a sponge, soaking up everything, and your conscious mind didn't possess the wisdom to distinguish between positive and negative data. It accepted both, and the more it was repeated, the more firmly it became embedded in your subconscious, where it turned into beliefs. Positive statements became positive beliefs. Negative statements became negative or faulty beliefs. However, you computed and responded to both, whether they were accurate or not. Your mind stored them away, deep in the subconscious.

Then again, perhaps you came from a household where every night you were told to "clean the plate because other children in the world are starving!" To this day you may not leave the table without finishing everything on your plate, even though as a mature, thinking adult, you know that "cleaning the plate" does nothing to feed starving children anywhere. Nevertheless, you shovel away every scrap of food because of some past faulty programming.

Not only were you programmed verbally, but you were conditioned in certain ways, too. For example, examine how food may have become important in your life. As a child, you fell and bruised your knee and went home crying. Mother comforted you, wiped away the tears, applied a Band-Aid, and soothed your pain with a nice big cookie! The association was made: Relief from pain = food! You computed that fast! So,

Beyond the Diet Syndrome 45

next time you got hurt, you looked for more than just Mother and a Band-Aid; you also needed and wanted the rest of the cure—food! This conditioning may have been reinforced every time you went to the family doctor, who administered your vaccination and then stopped the tears with a lollipop!

Thus you learned early that food relieves pain. Eating made you feel better; and simultaneously, of course, this was being programmed into your mind for some future *misuse*. When you've been programmed to believe food is the panacea for all ills, the results can prove devastating. Such was the case with Helen, a former student and one of my favorite M.I.N.D. OVER WEIGHT® success stories.

When Helen first came to see me, she was a 19-year-old college student who weighed 225 pounds and was 5 feet 6 inches tall. She was an intelligent girl who had become expert at the diet game, vowing to herself each time that she was going to lose weight and keep it off, only to find herself failing time after time. In her eyes, her entire life was falling apart. She felt as though she were destined to be overweight forever. What else was there to her life, except the diet syndrome?

An only child who lived at home with her adoring parents, she was so obsessed with the constant fear of being overweight that her school work deteriorated and her social life became restricted to watching television in her room while eating anything available.

Helen's parents became desperate. Here was their only child, a lovely, intelligent young woman, whose entire life revolved around food, and whose compulsion to eat was ruining her life. They loved her dearly, but they were heartsick. So they became her keepers—the keepers of her diet, that is—often conducting unannounced searches for contraband food in her bedroom at midnight. On occasion, they caught her before she got to the food and were able to confiscate it. Most of the time they were too late; the only evidence that Helen had been sneak-eating was the empty candy-bar wrappers.

In the beginning, to teach her how to use the M.I.N.D. OVER WEIGHT® method, I convinced her that she wasn't doomed to be fat for the rest of her life, and that she wouldn't have to go on a diet. I showed her she had to concentrate on the Method to alter her faulty belief that she would always have a weight problem. And that's exactly what M.I.N.D. OVER WEIGHT® did for her. It helped her achieve a better understanding of herself and her weight problem so that she could solve it. Ironically, we discovered that Helen's parents were at the root of her faulty overweight belief. They had always expressed their love for her with exotic foods and elaborate desserts, prepared lovingly by Helen's father, whose hobby was gourmet cooking. Not an outgoing child, she would stay home nights helping her parents prepare the evening's culinary delights. She enjoyed participating in and sampling all the pleasures of her parents' hobby. After all, it was a lot of fun to get together and prepare exciting new recipes every night—more fun than going out with her friends.

As time went on, Helen became the family's official food taster. It gave her a great deal of pleasure to see her parents smiling with approval every time she proclaimed, "The food's ready. It tastes perfect. Let's eat!" The approval of her parents encouraged her to stay home more and more. Because food was the center of their universe, it became the source of Helen's contentment. If she was unhappy, food eased the pain; if she was ill, food made her feel better; if she was frightened, food gave her strength. Mealtimes were the happiest times, no matter what had happened during the day. She always knew that her solace was on the kitchen table. Unwittingly, her parents were reinforcing the belief that food represented security, safety, and love.

This programmed pattern of Helen's life-style continued throughout her school years. By the time she got to college, she was extremely overweight. The happy family hobby had turned into a nightmare! Finally, when her parents realized that Helen's over-eating was a compulsion seemingly out of control, they abandoned the exotic cuisine and the nightly rituals of food preparation. Not surprisingly, Helen felt threatened by this; it was her greatest happiness, and they were taking it away. She loved her parents dearly and wanted to please them, but she couldn't give up her happiness... and happiness, to her, focused on food! So she took to following strict diets in front of them, while becoming a sneak-eater.

The deceptions she perpetrated caused her to feel intolerably guilty. She was hurting the people she loved most in the world—her parents. She felt responsible for their misery. She couldn't endure the agony she saw in their eyes and felt helpless to change it into the loving approval she used to see there. Unable to stop, her self-image battered, she drove herself to eat still more because her mind had been programmed to believe that food always eased pain. Of course, she gained even more weight. She was trapped in a vicious cycle, and the drama of the diet syndrome, because of early faulty beliefs that had been programmed into her subconscious mind.

How have you been programmed for overweight?

Perhaps you come from an overweight family. Your parents or your brothers and sisters might be overweight, and you grew up in an environment in which the major topic of conversation for the household was food. And when you weren't talking about it, you were eating it. In fact, your earliest memories of family get-togethers might be of mealtimes—these large people gathered around a dining-room table devouring great quantities of food. Of course, you were encouraged and expected to follow suit.

Bob, another M.I.N.D. OVER WEIGHT® success story, came from such an environment. Dinner for his family was always a four-hour, eleven-course gluttony. Meals of swinish size were normal to Bob. In fact, it wasn't until he was twelve years old that he realized that everyone didn't eat the way his family did. While visiting some friends, he discovered that their families did other things Sundays beside eat. By then, Bob weighed 150 pounds and stood 4 feet 11 inches tall. His own family had added permanent insult to his overweight injury by nicknaming him "Big Bob!" It's not hard to imagine what his developing self-image was like.

As he matured, he was bombarded with statements such as, "You're not fat, you've got big bones!" and "There's nothing you can do about it, you're built like your father!" By the time he was 15, he'd been told many times that he was going to be overweight because "it ran in the family." Once it became a belief, buried deep in his subconscious, his mind had been programmed to accept the fact that there was an overweight body in his future. He'd been programmed not only to accept it, but to expect it!

Think about it...

The first time one of your own school friends teasingly called you Fatso, a little voice in the back of your mind whispered, "Uh oh, it really is happening." You probably ran home, looked in the mirror, and imagined you saw the extra poundage, but weren't sure. So you anxiously asked your parents, "Am I getting fat?" "Well, dear," came the probable answer, "at this age, you should be filling out anyway."

That's all your young subconscious had to near! You didn't have a weight problem as yet, but you were being told that when you reached a certain age, you had to *expect* to gain weight. Naturally, your mind will manifest that belief in your body by directing you to eat more. Sooner or later, you will have a weight problem. You *expect* it to happen, so it will.

Another case of copycatting bad nutritional behavior occurs when you're programmed to imitate the behavior of a frustrated dieter, a person who diets, cheats on diets, and breaks diets time and again. For example, imagine what must go through the mind of a child the first time he's aware that his mother is caught up in the diet syndrome. When he comes home from school, he's used to having a snack. However, one day he goes to the cookie jar and finds it empty! When he asks for cookies, he is informed there will be no more cookies in the house because Mother's decided she's put on too much weight and has started a diet.

Cookies and milk after school is a habit difficult for a youngster to break, so every day the child keeps checking the jar, only to be disappointed. Now he's really confused. His mother's the one who's over-weight. Not him. Why can't he have any cookies? Finally he asks for an explanation. She tells him that she has to lose weight and can't eat cookies because they're fattening. Therefore, she won't have them in the house.

The child watches his mother diet for six straight days. He knows she's still on a diet because the cookie jar remains empty. He also knows that his mother has been irritable, short-tempered, and angry with every-one in the household. So the connection is made: Mommy's unhappy when she *can't* have cookies.

Is it surprising then, when the child comes home from school on the seventh day and notices that the cookie jar is filled and his mother is happy and smiling, that he concludes having cookies makes Mommy happy? Of course not. The child's conscious mind connects both situations and comes out with a new piece of data, a new belief programmed into his subconscious: Food makes people happy. Therefore, food will make him happy, too.

By now you don't have to guess what's going to happen to this child. With this newfound belief, rein-forced again and again by watching his mother suffer while she struggles to get thin, he's bound to assume the fat role one day. In his own quest for happiness, he's going to eat a lot of food and become overweight.

•

Your own self-image is created by all the beliefs you have about yourself and your world. Some of those beliefs are faulty, giving you a distorted view of yourself and reinforcing a poor self-image instead of a positive, strong concept. When you're dealing with overweight, the self-image usually ends up battered and bruised. After you've overindulged in eating, the old programming comes flooding back. It only takes a quick glance in the mirror to observe a few new bulges on the body of that overweight person staring back to strengthen your faulty overweight beliefs. You start reinforcing it in your subconscious mind through your conscious thoughts. You do it with statements like "It's not my fault, I just don't burn up food as fast as other people do!" or "I can't control myself" or "I'm always going to be overweight, just like my mother!" And so on and so on.

Is it any wonder why you have problems keeping weight off? You're still accepting overweight as an inevitable fact of life. Every time you try another diet, you prove it to yourself all over again. You go along, doing great for one or two weeks, and then one day you reach for a cookie. It's quite a normal thing for other people to do—but not for you. You're different. You have a weight problem. But you eat anyway until it strikes you. You blew it again. You're so *bad*. You have no *control*, no *will power*.

Binge time! There goes the *whole box* of cookies. Why not? You can't stick to a diet. You always fail. You'll never be thin.

How many times has this happened to you?

Every time it happens, it merely reinforces the overweight pattern that keeps you trapped in the diet syndrome.

Think about it...

What makes you go on an uncontrollable eating binge? When do you overeat?

Try this simple little multiple-choice test by filling in the blank.

"I overeat when I feel _____ *"*

a. *angry*   g. *inadequate*

b. *nervous*   h. *insecure*

c. *anxious*   i. *bored*

d. *depressed*   j. *frightened*

e. *upset*   k. *all of the above*

f. *guilty*

These are a few of the self-programmed trigger mechanisms that send you on a mad dash to the refrigerator or a wild drive to the candy store. It happens this way because you've been programmed in the past to believe that food makes you feel better. Food is love. Food is security. Food relieves anxiety. It helps you cope with life better. In fact, food is one of the most important things in your life and you've never before known *why*. It's become a simple reflex action. When you feel "bad," you reach for food without even thinking about it.

Tension and anxiety are two of the other most common trigger mechanisms for overweight. After all, this is a very stressful and anxiety-ridden world. Perhaps it happens to you when stuck in a traffic jam. By the time you arrive at your destination, you have to calm your shattered nerves by devouring three dough-nuts before you finish your first cup of coffee. Why shouldn't you have those doughnuts? Look at all you went through! You deserve a little pleasure, don't you?

Or, after seeing the kids off to school, you find yourself utterly frustrated by the sight of all the messy breakfast dishes in the sink. So you soothe your frustra-tion with a slice of coffee cake. Why not? It made you feel better when you ate it yesterday morning...and the day before. Bingo! A new self-destructive program has been created!

Often the mere thought of having to start a diet will trigger you to eat. Actually, almost any anxiety-producing situation will send you to the nearest source of food. Most of the time you don't realize what—or how much—you've eaten until you've finished it!

It could be that other people trigger you to eat. That happened to Lisa, a career woman in her mid-twenties, who had been plagued for four years by an extra thirty pounds. Until she learned the M.I.N.D. OVER WEIGHT® method, she was never able to lose a single one of those pounds, no matter how hard she tried. In her case, the major trigger for her overeating was her mother. Lisa would visit weekly. As soon as she walked in the door, her mother would begin nagging her about her overweight problem, among other things. Lisa, like a robot, was programmed to run directly to the refrigerator, where, in defiance, she ate everything within reach for the duration of the visit.

Her revenge was always short-lived. As soon as Lisa left her mother's house and got into her car, the guilt would set in. By the time she got home, she would be so furious at herself and her lack of control that she would head for the bathroom, stick her fingers down her throat, and throw up. By the time she came to see me, this vicious cycle had been going on for years. Moreover, Lisa was no longer maintaining her weight at the thirty pounds over where she wanted it to be; she was *gaining*. Such is the destructive power of trigger mechanisms.

Your own weight problem might be a fairly recent one. Only lately have a few extra pounds begun to plague you. There might not appear to be any reason for your sudden weight gain, but you can be sure there is. It's been my experience to recognize a similar pattern in almost every case. Although the situations were different, the results were always the same. A weight gain happened because of a faulty belief, like the widespread belief that if you stop smoking you will gain weight. It's not necessary; you just *expect* it to happen. The truth is that most people who give up smoking *do* gain weight, since they've programmed themselves into believing they will.

Another faulty belief is the one that supposes "when you reach a certain age, you should expect to gain weight because your metabolism has slowed down." You may have tucked that one away, deep in your subconscious. Unless your physician has confirmed this to be a medical problem, then your sudden weight gain is merely a faulty belief manifesting itself in your body.

Some people even accidentally program themselves to gain weight. Tell yourself that you'll gain a pound if you eat that slice of lemon meringue pie; as long as you believe it, you will indeed put on a pound.

That is the darker side of the power of belief.

Think about it...

Your mind has been successfully programmed for the overweight role. And as long as you continue to feed its faulty inner beliefs with repetitive, negative thoughts, it will keep your body in an overweight condition no matter what external methods you try.

What is important is how you view yourself. If you believe you'll never be anything but overweight, you'll never be thin. Have you ever thought that you weren't *born* programmed to believe you had to be overweight? You programmed yourself to believe it, and you let other people do it to you. What's worse, you didn't even know it was happening to you at the time. *Now* you know, and you *can* do something about it.

You can change your programming.

The tool you will use is your own mind. It's more powerful than any computer ever devised. It takes its direction from you. You can reprogram it any way you want. You've dreamed of being able to sit in a restaurant and order whatever you wanted without considering whether or not it was "fattening." You've yearned for the time when food would simply be a part of your life—something you would think about when you were hungry, and not an enemy with which to do battle every waking moment. You would love to say to your host or hostess when they offer you second helpings of dessert after a big meal, "No, thanks, I don't want any more"—and *really mean it!*

In other words, your deepest desire is to be able to decide for yourself what to eat, how much to eat, and when to eat without supervision from anything or anybody outside of yourself.

You can do it. It's not an impossible dream. There is a way to a thinner you by a better understanding of yourself through the M.I.N.D. OVER WEIGHT® method that will take you beyond the diet syndrome to a happy, thin life.

Chapter 3
LIGHTEN UP

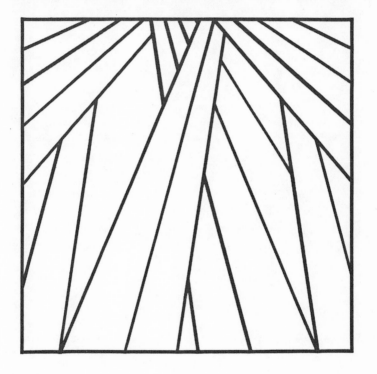

You're really going to enjoy "lightening up." It's like taking your own mini-vacation—a vacation where you can "get away from it all" for a while, relax and let go of the anxieties of the overweight drama; where you can be alone with yourself and enjoy the pleasure of your own company; where you can experience peace and health, and think about yourself for a change. Lightening up is a wonderfully elevating experience, one that will give your spirits a lift. It's the first part of the M.I.N.D. OVER WEIGHT® method.

Several things will happen. The first thing you'll learn to do is relax yourself—to relax your body *and* your mind. Once you're completely relaxed, both physically and mentally, you'll come to a better understanding of how your mind and body work together. In this way, you'll be put in touch with your subconscious mind, the place where you'll be able to find and change the faulty beliefs that are preventing you from becoming the thin person you want to be.

What follows are your directions for doing Part One of the M.I.N.D. OVER WEIGHT® method. Read through all of the instructions completely. Don't try to read and practice them at the same time. Read each direction carefully. Familiarize yourself with each step along the way, and prepare yourself for a very pleasant experience.

Choose a quiet place where you can be alone, a peaceful place where you'll be undisturbed for about ten minutes. (If all else fails in your search for a "quiet place" the bathroom is always a good choice.)

Sit comfortably upright, either in your favorite chair or on the floor. If you choose a chair, keep both feet flat on the floor. Don't cross your legs or ankles. If you prefer to sit on the floor, you may brace your back against the wall. Your legs may be either crossed or straight out in front of you. Let your body settle in for a few seconds.

Sit with your hands on your lap.
Then gently close your eyes.

1

Now, gently, take a deep breath.
Imagine the breath going all the way to the very top of your head, and hold it there.
Hold the breath there for a moment.
Think about it.
Become aware of it.
Experience it.
And, very gently, as you exhale, imagine the breath passing all the way down through your body, beginning to relax it.
Feel your body begin to relax.

Repeat these slow, deep breaths three or four times.
Then breathe normally.

2 _____

Now, gently, bring your attention to your scalp.
Think about your scalp.
Concentrate on it.
Become aware of it.
And, in your mind, imagine your scalp relaxing.
Think of it relaxing.
And let it relax.

3 _____

Now, gently, bring your attention to your forehead.
Think about your forehead.
Concentrate on it.
Become aware of it. Experience it.
Be gentle.
Now let your forehead relax.
Let it relax completely.

4 _____

Now, gently, bring your attention to your eyelids.
Think about your eyelids.
Sense them and feel them.
Become aware of the presence of your eyelids.
Acknowledge them. Experience them.
And let your eyelids relax.
Let them relax ... and feel them relax.

5 _____

Now, gently, bring your attention to your cheeks and your jawbone.

Think about your cheeks and your jawbone.

Feel them and sense them.

Now, with your mind, relax your cheeks and jawbone completely.

Let them relax and notice them relaxing.

As your body relaxes, notice that your mind becomes very calm and very peaceful.

And notice that you are in control of your mind and your body.

6 _____

Now, gently, think about your throat and the back of your neck.

Become aware of them in your mind.

Feel them.

Sense them.

Experience them.

Now let your throat and the back of your neck relax.

Let them relax completely.

7

Now, gently, bring your attention to your shoulders,
your arms, and your hands.
Imagine them.
Feel them.
See them clearly in your mind.
And let them relax.
Relax your shoulders,
your arms,
and your hands
completely.

8

Now, gently, become aware of your chest.
Feel it slowly rising and falling,
rising and falling.
Follow the rhythm of your chest.
Experience it.
Now, while breathing naturally, relax your chest area
completely.
Let your chest relax.

Notice that your body is relaxing and that your mind is
becoming calm and clear.

9 _____

Now, gently, bring your attention to the small of your back and your stomach.
Think about them.
See them in your mind.
Become aware of them.
Become aware of your stomach and the small of your back.
Feel them and sense them.
And let them relax.
Let your stomach and your back relax.

10 _____

Now, bring your awareness to your buttocks and your hips.
Feel the pressure of your buttocks against the chair or floor.
Feel and experience your hips.
Become aware of your buttocks and your hips.
Think about them.
Sense them.
And let them relax.
Let them relax completely and feel them relax.

11 _____

Now, gently, think about your thighs and the calves of your legs.
Become aware of them.
Sense them.
Feel them.
Experience their presence.
And let them relax, now.
Relax your thighs and the calves of your legs completely.

12 _____

Now, gently, bring your attention to your feet.
Feel them touching the floor.
Become aware of them.
Think about them.
Experience them.
And let your feet relax.
Let them relax completely.
And feel them relax.

Notice how relaxed your body is. Notice how calm and clear your mind is.

Realize that you are in complete control of your mind and your body at all times.

13 _____

Now, gently, bring your attention to the tip of your nose, to your nostrils.
Become aware of the breath as it comes in and goes out of the nostrils.
Concentrate on the tip of your nose.
Notice the breath coming in and going out.
Don't follow the breath into your body.
Just watch the breath gently entering and leaving the nostrils.

If a thought comes into your mind, acknowledge the thought and then let it go *by bringing your attention back to the breath at the nostrils.*

Any time a thought comes into your mind, don't block it.
Acknowledge the thought and let it go, simply by bringing your attention back to the breath as it gently enters and leaves your nostrils.

Continue to watch the breath in this manner for at least three minutes.

Then gently open your eyes.

What you have just read is Part One of the M.I.N.D. OVER WEIGHT® method. Now I would like you to experience it. Go back and reread the text several times. It is designed to be easy to remember. Once you know the steps, consider the next ten minutes as your own little mini-vacation. Put the book down and do Part One of the Method. Then come back.

•

Wasn't that nice?

For the past ten minutes, you have been in complete control of your mind and your body. And you did it yourself! Think about how good you feel now. Do you notice how relaxed you are? How peaceful you feel? How clear your mind is? How calm your body? Notice that there is no tension in your body and no anxiety in your mind. When was the last time you felt this relaxed?

You will find as you continue to practice this part of the Method, you'll be more relaxed more of the time, and that your mind will be much clearer.

There are three different techniques involved in Part One of the Method that must be examined more closely so you understand the reasons behind them and how they work. First, doing the deep. slow breathing is an age-old remedy to release tension. Do you remember the adage that tells you to take a deep breath and count to ten when you feel the need to calm down? It worked then, and it works now. It's a good beginning to total relaxation.

Secondly, doing the step-by-step relaxation of the parts of your body trains your mind to control your body and to relax it at will. Your mind is a powerful entity, and you can use it in this manner to consciously relieve your body of tension and anxiety. You don't need a hot bath, a pill, or a whipped-cream cake to calm yourself; you can use your mind to do it.

And finally, the technique of watching the breath helps you develop mental discipline. By giving yourself the focal point of the breath *at the nostrils*, you're keeping your attention on a single activity, which serves to calm the busy, cluttered thoughts of your conscious mind. In effect, you are choosing what to think about, what to concentrate on. You are in the process of developing a calm, clear space in your mind—a space that you will be using in Part Two of the M.I.N.D. OVER WEIGHT® method to achieve a permanently thin body.

In just ten minutes of lightening up you have become more in touch with your own body, more aware of how it works, more conscious of the relationship of your body to your mind. Most importantly, you have accomplished some sense of being more in control.

Don't you already feel better about yourself?

Think about it...

You can feel this good about yourself every day by practicing the Method. The more you practice, the better you'll feel. It's best to set aside some time each morning to practice before the day begins. If you can't do it then, it's fine to practice anytime you wish except late at night. After the deep relaxation of Part One of the Method, you'll find your energy level has been renewed and you'll be wide awake. The only time not recommended is before bedtime.

Practice ought to occur at the same time every day so that doing the Method becomes an established part of your daily routine, like washing your face or brushing your teeth. Moreover, if you feel drowsy during your first attempts, don't be concerned—it's perfectly normal. After all, you're not accustomed to being this relaxed. The drowsiness stage will pass quickly.

Furthermore, you should not lie down when you're practicing the Method. Rather, sit in an upright position. This will enhance your increased awareness and your ability to use your mind more clearly, both of which are necessary. If you find yourself slouching over as you proceed with the techniques, simply place your hands, palms up, on your lap. This will keep your shoulders back and will prevent you from slouching.

If the phone rings or you are distracted in any way while practicing, stop and take care of the interruption. Then resume your practice from where you left off. Remember, you are always in control.

By all means, don't be afraid to move, if you must. I've known many people who suffered through the entire Method with an unbearably itchy nose. It's okay to scratch your nose if it itches. After a while, though, you won't be bothered by any distractions of the body.

However, you may find that you are most often distracted by inner thoughts, especially when you are first learning to master the watching-the-breath technique. This, too, is a common occurrence. Bear with it for a while. Simply bring your attention back to the breath at the nostrils. As you become more experienced in the use of this technique, you'll find yourself being less and less bothered by distracting thoughts welling to the surface of your consciousness.

Part One of the Method has brought you to what I will characterize as a higher level of consciousness. It enables you to *consciously* use more of your mind more of the time. In time, you won't have to do the technique of relaxing each part of your body separately, because by then you will have learned how to relax your entire body at one time, at will.

Learning to use your mind is like learning to ride a bicycle for the first time. You don't just mount a bike and race away like a champion first time out. Someone has to teach you the basics. Your own initial attempts at it were probably clumsy, but each time you practiced, you got better, until one day you did it effortlessly. So it is with this part of the M.I.N.D. OVER WEIGHT® method. Relax and enjoy the experience of lightening up. The more often you do it, the sooner you'll have a better understanding of yourself through an expanded self-awareness. This technique prepares the way for you to get in touch with your subconscious mind—the place where you will be able to challenge and revise your faulty overweight beliefs, and where you will change the mental picture of yourself into a slim one.

Chapter 4

M.I.N.D.
OVER
WEIGHT®

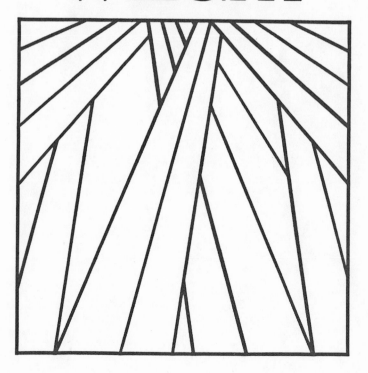

How many times have you heard the statement "Think slim and you'll lose weight"? Somehow you knew it made sense; the problem was making it work. If you did manage to think slim, you probably could not sustain it for any extended period of time. This happened because it was a concept too much on the surface of your mind, easily dismissed by the reality of the overweight drama you were living. However, now that you've lightened up, you will find it easier going.

Part Two of the Method will make thinking slim happen to you naturally—on more than the surface level of your mind. You'll begin to *believe* it in your subconscious as well by setting to work changing negative thoughts and beliefs into positive ones. This will take place on both levels of consciousness, by using conscious thoughts to direct subconscious functions. On this higher-level consciousness you will begin to implant the new programming of M.I.N.D. OVER WEIGHT®. The process resembles taking your own photograph, with your mind serving as the camera lens. In a state of total relaxation, you will see yourself thin, and click!—you will superimpose a newer image onto your subconscious.

How does this develop into the finished product? The major ingredient is your imagination. It is important to realize that imagination is the essence of all creation. Everything begins as a thought, an idea. The table at which you eat, the chair in which you sit, the bed on which you sleep—all began as abstractions in someone's mind before they could be manufactured. Each emerged as an idea that soon solidified into a mental picture, an imaginary concept. Then it was transferred onto a drawing board, in the form of a blueprint to be produced for use.

Think about it....

You are going to learn how to design the mental blueprint for your perfect, slim body. You will use your imagination to seed your mind. With this part of the Method, you will also be able to change the faulty overweight beliefs you hold about yourself into healthy, thin ones.

What follows are the steps for Part Two of the Method. Familiarize yourself with them by reading the written instructions before you begin the Method, as you did in Chapter 3.

1 _____

Repeat Part One of the Method:
Take three or four deep breaths
Relax your body
Watch the breath

Instead of opening your eyes, continue with the following steps, filling the space you have cleared in your mind.

2 _____

Sit quietly.

In your mind imagine a mist, a swirling white mist.

As you look at the mist, imagine the image of yourself emerging slowly.

As the mist clears away, see the image of yourself getting thinner and thinner. Getting thinner as you watch.

Concentrate on the image of the perfect you.

See how slim and attractive you are.

Notice how happy you are.

3

Ever so gently, imagine merging with this image of the perfect you.

In your mind, become it now.

Merge with the new image of yourself.

Feel the fulfillment of having attained your desired size.

Experience the satisfaction of being this thin you, this new you.

4

Imagine moving around in this slim, healthy body.
Experience the lightness of your body.
In your mind, move around in this perfect body.
Feel the ease with which you move.
Imagine bending over, touching your toes.
Feel how easy it is.
Imagine sitting down in a chair. Cross your legs.
Feel and imagine the pleasure of this.
Feel how slim your body is.
Experience these pleasant emotions.
Experience it, feel it, become it.
Know the happiness that is yours at this moment.

5 _____

Imagine looking into a mirror.

Turn to each side.

See your slim profile.

Imagine wearing your favorite style of clothes.

Notice how attractive you are.

Feel the fulfillment of this achievement. Your perfect size.

Sense it, feel it, imagine it.

Spend a few moments in this space. Peaceful. Calm. Clear. Relaxed.

Experience yourself with this slim, attractive figure.

Know that it is yours.

Know that it is always yours.

This is you. This is the real you.

Free of excess pounds.

Free of the burden of being overweight.

See it in your mind. Feel it in your mind.

Experience the happiness of this achievement.

Bringing these feelings with you, gently open your eyes.

Now put the book down, and do the entire Method in sequence—Part One and Part Two.

•

Reflect on the entire Method itself. Didn't it feel wonderful to experience the joy of being thin? Wasn't it a grand feeling to know you were in control of your body and mind? You can experience this peaceful, calm knowledge every day. Ultimately, as it becomes real in your mind, it will become real in your life! *Believe* it!

You'll notice that Part Two of the Method contained a series of progressive visualizations and emotional experiences you followed.

You first experienced the "clear space" in your mind, which you did to get in touch with subconscious areas—beyond the restrictions of the conscious mind, a space where you are free of doubt, anxiety, and fear. This was necessary so that your perspective on reality could expand.

Imagination became the vehicle used to harness the power of your mind, and positive emotions the fuel to propel new mental pictures into the subconscious. The mist technique was used as a starting point to set your imagination into gear and working for you. Seeing yourself emerge from the mist gave you the opportunity to create and solidify the mental picture of the desired thin body you want to have.

In merging with the image of the perfect you, you started to experience the *feelings* of having a thin body. Moving around in this thin body, in your mind, taught you to live as though you were already thin, building upon that mental experience with the daily practice of reinforcing those feelings. This technique was fashioned to assist you in living a thin life even before you achieve your thin body in actuality, accustoming yourself to a thin life *mentally*, and setting the mood for a thin reality.

Seeing yourself in the mirror gave you the fulfillment of seeing this achievement, of admiring the results of your efforts, of knowing the satisfaction that the end result will bring you.

In the last step of the Method, you spent a few moments immersing yourself in the wonderful emotions of being thin, experiencing fully the happiness you felt as a thin person. This is an important step, because emotions are very powerful. They send this new image into your subconscious, and add power to your new belief in yourself as a thin person.

In sum, using the Method puts you in touch with your subconscious mind, enabling you to implant the picture and feelings of the thin you. Because the subconscious is open to your control in this clear space, it will accept what you give to it, as the subconscious is neutral territory. It doesn't reason things out, or question why material is being fed into it—it simply produces whatever it is instructed. Furthermore, it doesn't judge between reality and imagination, because they are both the same in the subconscious dominion. This is the very reason why it accepted all the faulty programming from your past. However, by using the Method you dislodge and expel faulty beliefs by creating and experiencing your desired end result in your mind, thus reversing the process that created the problem in the first place.

Regular practice will insure that the memory of the thin you that you experienced is strongly embedded in your subconscious. It is in this way that you will take charge of your mental patterns and your life as a thin person.

It's not unusual to hear beginning students of M.I.N.D.® say:

"I get distracted when I'm practicing the Method."

"I don't think I can do it, because there are too many things on my mind. I find myself thinking of whom I must call, or shopping, or repairing the car, or mowing the lawn, and so on."

"I can't seem to get to the point where my mind is absolutely clear."

If you find yourself wandering in this fashion, take a few extra deep breaths. This will help to calm your body and enable you to focus your mind on each succeeding step of the Method. You're most likely to run into some conscious resistance when you are at the point in Part One of the Method of "watching the breath." If this happens, you might find it helpful to count the breaths from one to ten several times, or repeat, "in breath, out breath" for a while. Give yourself a few days to perfect the technique of concentration.

If you're having any trouble imagining yourself as thin in Part Two of the Method, it's only because you have to understand that "seeing" while you're doing the Method is not the same as seeing something with your eyes. In your mind, you merely conjure the desired image, but mental pictures are not as clear as sighted pictures. At first the vision may appear out of focus. If you think you can't visualize properly, concentrate on the ideal you. Soon you *will* see it, not only in your mind, but on your body as well.

•

The power of belief and imagination has propelled ordinary people to accomplish incredible goals. Two bicycle repairmen named Wright used to fantasize about flying like birds. It started them thinking: "Could we build a machine that would fly?"The idea captured their imaginations, and they continued to daydream about it. They imagined themselves flying like the birds they carefully studied. These mental experiences became so real to them, they began to believe they could build such a machine; so they continued to work, directed by this mental picture which ultimately became the first flying machine.

It may appear simplistic to state a single example of the creative use of the imagination in this manner, but the mechanisms of the mind operate in this basic and powerful way.

The great masters of music, art, and science share a common quality—the ability to create something real out of imagination and belief. You are no different! You have the same capacity to create your own slim *reality* by using your mind to revise faulty beliefs. By regularly utilizing this power to become what you want to be, you can mold your thoughts and beliefs and impress them with the positive emotions of being thin. Soon your mind will manifest these feelings into a slim body.

In Part One you learned how to control your body. Part Two enabled you to control not only your body, but your mind. You chose healthy, positive thoughts, sending them into your subconscious, programming yourself with a slim mental picture, and establishing healthy beliefs about yourself—in effect, designing a new self-image. The calm, clear, open mind achieved in Part One permitted this constructive work to be done. Into this "calm space" of a cleared subconscious, you designed the changes that must be made in your body. You visualized yourself as you are going to be— slim, peaceful, and happy. Then, in your mind, you merged into the perfect you. Doing this made it possible for you to experience—with all its consequent emotions and feelings—what being naturally thin is really like.

Experience means more than just the things you go through in life, just as *merging* the image of the old you with the perfect you means more than observing it. The difference is as great as admiring a beautiful new car and actually getting into it, feeling the wheel beneath your hands, and driving it. Experience must encompass the *feelings* you have in your mental life, with all its hopes and wishes.

In this perspective, examine how *real* was the experience of being thin in your mind. The experience you gained conceptualizing something *with emotion and belief* has the same value *to your mind* as if you had experienced the physical reality. Your mental experience has the same *impact* as a life experience. It has the same *value* to both your conscious and subconscious mind.

Was this some magician's trick, deceiving the mind in this way? Not at all; you were simply exercising part of the ability you always possessed within you. Clearly, if the mind has the capacity to store, repress, and regenerate negative or faulty beliefs, doesn't it follow that the same is true of positive beliefs that can elevate and enrich your life?

The stage is now set for your success.

Imagining yourself as a slim person—at a higher level of consciousness—will not only give you the *feeling* of being thin, but the *knowledge* that it is real, that it is *possible* for you to accomplish it.

Becoming a thin person must start in your mind, since it is the drawing board for your subconscious. Here you devise the blueprints for the finished product. This time you are assured it is your *own* creation.

You are the creator of your body.

You imagine yourself slim and healthy.

Your mind will produce the desired, believed-in result.

Chapter 5

FREE AT LAST! STOP DIETING

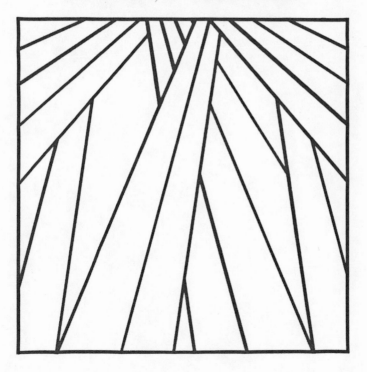

Now you can stop the diet merry-go-round. Say farewell to the unpleasant routine of looking for another new diet. You can enjoy a different kind of diet. Using the Method every day is a *mental* diet. It is one that eliminates the usual stress and strain associated with ordinary weight-loss programs. Diet regimens aren't designed to make you feel peaceful and calm; in fact, they *create* more stress and anxiety. Think about the enormous pressure the diet discipline placed on you. You were always frightened of the moment when you would break your diet, and this constant anxiety became your daily companion. You woke every morning with thoughts such as, "I've got to stick to my diet today. This time, I must make it." There was no peace. No relief. The pressure was on: worrying about what to eat and what not to eat. It became a continuous struggle. You don't *need* it anymore.

More importantly, dieting reinforced the faulty belief that you were overweight by *confirming* that self-image; that is, to diet meant that you must be overweight. Being a dieter kept you stuck in the "fat role."

Now you've taken the first step to change roles. You're writing a thin "script" for yourself. You've discovered the formula for permanent weight loss, working from the inside out, not from the outside in. Diets won't accomplish what you want because they are not designed to change your thinking or beliefs about yourself. The Method helps you change your beliefs and thinking, altering the mental picture you have of yourself. Your self-image is a direct result of your thoughts and beliefs, and since your body reflects self-image, using the Method to make these inner changes eliminates the need for diets.

Your *daily use* of the Method will teach you to use more of your mind more of the time. After all, having an expanded self-awareness simply means using more of your mind on a conscious level. The Method proves that you are in control of your mind and your body, and being in control of your mind and body means being in control of your life.

Start by trusting yourself, and watch your lifestyle change. You'll feel good about yourself. You'll be much more aware of your better qualities, those that got buried in the diet drama. And, after a week or two of using the Method, you'll notice a subtle change in your eating habits. You'll start to eat the way a thin person eats. You'll find yourself eating what you want, when you want, but in *quantities* of food appropriate to a thin person. You won't have to refuse food you want, because you won't want the amounts of food you used to. You will no longer fear food, because it is going to take its proper place in your life.

In a larger sense, the Method is a logical, practical application of your ability to take charge of your body by taking charge of your mind. It is a process that simply requires practice and perseverance in following its techniques.

•

Rich, a recent student of M.I.N.D. OVER WEIGHT®, had a severe weight problem. Seemingly, he had no control over his eating habits. He ate once a day—*all* day long—and he had no idea what a "leftover" meant! This compulsive eating brought his weight to over three hundred pounds, and his health was endangered. I worked with him on his problem, and after working with the Method for a month, he was consuming three average meals a day with an evening snack. He told me that he was surprised to discover he hardly thought about food at all.

Even though he was still heavy at this time, he began to see himself as a thin person. So he ate like one. Rich never imagined he would want to refuse food. Now he does! Food is no longer the centerpiece of his life. His thoughts have turned toward career, his other goals in life, his happiness.

•

Jean, another M.I.N.D.® student, was more than a little surprised to find out the day she started the Method that there are *no forbidden foods*. It took her a while to stop laughing after I explained that there are no diets involved with M.I.N.D. OVER WEIGHT®. Still, I couldn't understand her wild laughter. She proceeded to relate to me her experience of the night before. ...

She was driving home from work, thinking about the new weight-loss program she was going to start the following day. As always, she wanted to have one last binge before her self-deprivation began. Naturally, she assumed that she would have to stop eating all the things she liked once she began the Method. Having been on and off diets for more than twenty years, she expected nothing else. She mulled over what she really wanted to have, settling on her favorite treat, ice-cream cake. Clutching the box in her hand, Jean went home and sat down to devour the entire cake.

It's clear to me now why she laughed so hard. She later confessed to me, "If I had known there were no forbidden foods, I would have eaten a little cake each night of the week. I didn't have to finish it at one sitting!"

After several months on the Method, she's doing

well, having lost thirty-four pounds. She still laughs at
the memory of her last binge!

•

Elaine, another success, recently enjoyed her first hot
fudge sundae in years. She adored hot fudge sundaes,
but they had always been one of the villains in her
overweight drama, so she had sworn off them years
before. Can you imagine her surprise, her joy, as she
savored each delicious spoonful? What made her
happiness complete was the knowledge that she
would no longer feel compelled to order a second
sundae five minutes after eating the first, as she had in
the past. Now she may have a hot fudge sundae if she
wishes, without feeling the old guilt about breaking a
diet. As a result, she views her life differently, enjoying
it more than before. It is not a bleak, dreary existence
of survival on diet foods, and anxiety-filled days, but a
healthy, full life-style that *includes* her favorite foods.
She is doing all this while losing weight steadily at the
rate of eight to ten pounds a month.

•

Laura's friends and coworkers noticed a distinct
change in her temperament shortly after she began to
practice the Method, and people began to remark
about these changes. When she first came to see me,
she was not only overweight, but extremely high-
strung and anxious. Interestingly, after using the
Method for three weeks, she became the office media-
tor—quite a different role for her. She was calmer and
more clearheaded because she was more in touch
with herself and her capabilities. Taking the fifteen-
minute mini-vacation every day resulted in an imme-
diate lessening in her tension and anxiety. Clearly, it

had proved its effectiveness, and for the first time in her life she was losing weight without stress.

These changes lent great support to Laura's new feelings of self-assurance and control. She is continually discovering nice qualities about herself that she hadn't been aware of for years.

•

Helen, our sneak-eater from Chapter 2, is one of my favorite success stories. She suffered from more than one agony with her overweight, but the changes in her that began to show within a few weeks of starting the Method were fantastic; not only did her midnight raids on the refrigerator cease, but the hidden caches of food in her room began to disappear. She ate average-sized meals with her family, while eliminating none of her favorites. Although at that time her weight still hovered around two hundred pounds, her attitude about herself began to reflect deep inner changes. She started to take an interest in her appearance, dressing in attractive clothes that didn't *necessarily* hide the overweight. This was her first step in accepting herself as she was.

Later, she acknowledged to me that because she accepted herself as she was, she started to care about herself. Such self-acceptance is important to becoming a slim person. For the first time in all her weight-losing years, Helen was getting thin *for herself*, not for someone else. She began to feel entitled to the happiness of being thin, and she began to express her independence, stand on her own, and achieve her full potential.

As this was happening, a mutual respect developed between her parents and Helen. She was growing with them in a mature way. Her parents stopped monitoring her food intake because she was taking charge of her own life. She made her own decisions about food and learned, with some surprise, how much self-control she had. She found her control *in her mind*, so that when her father offered her something he prepared, she could say "No, thanks," and he didn't feel hurt as before; he felt only admiration in seeing this new side of his daughter.

These changes occurred as Helen became aware of all the bad programming that had been locked in her subconscious. She was working with the Method to root out the old programming. As she succeeded in doing that, she found a unique, capable individual inside. Her self-image came around three hundred sixty degrees. Even before she reached her desired weight goal, Helen told me she liked what she saw in the mirror more than she had at points in her life when she was thinner. She came to understand this paradox. In the past, during her "thin times," she considered herself overweight no matter what she looked like.

Like Helen, you must *start accepting yourself as you are* without harsh self-judgments. *Don't* say you'll like yourself *when* you get thin. Start to like yourself *now* ... exactly as you are. This is the beginning of your successful thin future. It is an important step to take in the process of becoming thin. *Accept yourself.*

"Accept myself with the overweight?" you ask. "But if I accept myself with the overweight, then I'll never be able to lose it." On the contrary, it's the *only* way to succeed at weight loss. Self-acceptance.

Acceptance of yourself means you *care* about yourself. You can't change and improve yourself unless you care. Accept yourself in the same manner you accept those you love: your family, your friends, the other people in your life. You accept *them* with all their faults. You care about *them* in spite of their shortcomings; so start treating *yourself* the same way. Up to now you've been looking at your outer appearance and seeing only the overweight condition of your body, and unfairly judging yourself *as a person* because of it. This is wrong.

In this connection, let me tell you a story about a diamond. The diamond didn't emerge from the ground brilliantly cut to perfection, ready to be mounted in a piece of jewelry. It was dirty, dull, and shapeless. If it were lying on the sidewalk, you may have walked right past it, never knowing what it really was. It takes the vision of a diamond cutter to know what's inside. With special tools and carefully designed cuts, he releases what's inside: the perfect diamond. The diamond was always there, but it needed the expertise of his craftsmanship to cut away the excess and bring out the brilliance of the perfect stone.

Think of yourself as a diamond in the rough. You don't need an outside craftsman to shape it into perfection; you are your own artisan. You've always had the capability to become a slim person. What you didn't possess was the know-how needed to release that inner, thinner you. Now you have the knowledge; just as the diamond cutter applied his skills to the uncut diamond to release its beauty, you can apply your will to shape your new image with the power of your mind!

Changes like these will happen to you even while you're still in an overweight condition. Before you reach your ideal weight, the *fear* of overweight will disappear, since you won't consider being overweight a problem anymore. Imagine how you will feel when you start your day thinking slim, being confident about yourself, and going through the whole day without worrying about food. *Put your scales away.* You won't have to check your weight on the scales every morning, noon, and night! So don't use them for the time being.

Scales keep your thoughts focused on the problem. They become a measure of your worth, not your weight. If you don't lose pounds fast enough, the scale makes you believe you're not going to make it. If you lose a few pounds, it suggests that you'd better check again tomorrow to make certain you've kept them off. Thus, the scales ignite a daily crisis. Every time you step on them, your anxiety level rises. They are a constant reminder of your overweight condition, rather than the solution.

Move your consciousness away from the daily suspense of checking and re-checking the numbers on your scale by putting the machine in the closet. You seldom see what you want to see, anyway. So, put them away!

When you are practicing the Method, you are in a state of expanded awareness, or higher consciousness. It's at this level that you are able to go beyond the limitations and restrictions of the conscious mind, and enter the realm of the subconscious. The experience of higher consciousness produced by the Method is so powerful, so real, that it automatically expands your perceptions of yourself. You no longer see yourself as fat. In your mind, you see the "slim me"; you experience the powerful emotions of being thin and *feeling* thin in your mind. In time, these feelings will manifest as your slim, healthy body.

Henceforth, you won't be a slave to a past that kept you stuck in the diet syndrome. Now, the power of imagination and belief will free you from those bonds by creating a healthy life-style that is different from that of the past. Imagination gives you the perception, the feeling, and the experience of being thin, coupled with the ability to do what you want with your life and change those areas you want.

By seeing yourself thin at a higher level of consciousness you are creating a fresh mental blueprint for yourself, forming a thin image to carry around with you wherever you go. In a short while, you will *become* that thin picture, producing the thin body you've been striving for. Your body will have no choice but to accommodate these new beliefs and feelings. As you begin to see the thin you emerge, you'll discover that you have done away with all the old programming, those faulty beliefs that have lain trapped in your subconscious.

This mind-to-body process works like this: Imagine a garden. You want to grow marigolds in this garden, so you buy marigold seeds. Next, you choose the right place to plant them. You make certain that the seeds are nourished by sun and water so that they'll grow into healthy plants. You check regularly to keep them from being choked by weeds, and see to it that they are continuing to get all the necessary nourishment. Beyond that care and attention, you know that you will have beautiful marigolds one day.

Your mind resembles that fertile garden, with yourself as the master gardener. It will grow whatever you plant. All you must do is to plant the right thought—the thought of being thin—in the proper place: the subconscious. To this thought, you add the nourishment of belief, weeding out any doubts by using your imagination.

Do you recall the earlier analogy of the tree with the blocked root? If someone were to take the time and effort to dig up the ground and remove the strangulating rock, the root would start to function again. Unblocked, the buds of new growth would begin to blossom on what was once a dying branch. The Method enables you to achieve similar results with your overweight body. Your efforts toward a slimmer profile don't begin with diets. You must begin by digging out faulty beliefs, going below the surface of your mind into your subconscious. And when you remove limiting beliefs about yourself, you free yourself to grow, to progress, and ultimately to succeed in becoming and staying slim.

In practicing the Method each day, you are changing faulty beliefs such as "I'll always have a weight problem" into healthy beliefs like "I'll always have a slim body." By *experiencing* that slimness of form *in your mind*, you're planting in your subconscious new beliefs about yourself, accomplished through the visualizations and emotions stimulated by the Method. Thus, when you change the belief that "I'll always have a weight problem" to "I'll always be thin," you establish in your mind that you really *are* a thin person, thereby setting belief into action.

Making these inner changes takes less effort than is required during the agonizing hours you spent dieting. Think about it. Using the Method only takes a few pleasant minutes each day. The way you continue to think and believe about yourself will determine how your body looks and feels. The emphasis *must be* to change your faulty beliefs and consequently change your patterns of thinking. *Change* your attitude about yourself. *Change* your opinion of yourself. In short, *change your self-image* toward a healthier one.

A word of caution: You should be patient with yourself. Like the garden, change takes some time. *How much* time depends on you. I have worked with many people, and they have been quite successful using the Method to overcome a weight problem. You're no different from them. You have a perfect mind—a mind more than able to fulfill your need and desire to become thin. You know how successful you've been in acting out the overweight role with all of its anxieties; imagine the rewards of successfully acting out the thin role! You're entitled to live a thin life, and you deserve all the benefits that come with it. Continual practice will assure your own success.

So, forget the past.

It doesn't matter a great deal how many diets you've been on—and off! It's all in the past. It doesn't matter a bit. The only thing that matters now is what you think and believe.

Forget the bad memories.

All of those failures were experiences. Past experiences. They are useful only for pointing out mistakes. The past will help you recognize what *not* to do again.

Now that you can see how it all might have happened, stop blaming yourself for past failures— stop blaming others for your overweight problem. You are in control. Be glad that you discovered what you can do about it: You can break the vicious cycle; you can say good-bye to diets and misery. It's time to let go the past.

Doesn't it feel good to know you are finally running the show?

This is *the* important time in your life ... time to walk the thin line.

Chapter 6

WALKING THE THIN LINE

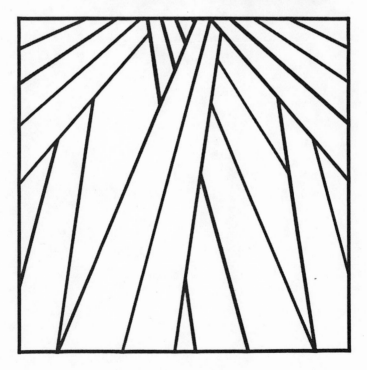

Ninety-five percent of people who lose weight soon gain it back, plus a couple of fresh pounds to heap insult onto injury. The only reason why lost weight returns is that you know you can't stay on diets forever. No one can suffer food deprivation for long. Having to live without the foods you enjoy prevents you from walking a thin line. Instead, you end up walking a tightrope. The common belief that you have to deprive yourself in order to have a thin body is the root cause of this needless suffering. But you needn't suffer in order to be thin, and the thought that the Method is *too easy to work* is not an unusual reaction.

Alan, a clinical psychologist, and a former student of M.I.N.D. OVER WEIGHT® (he lost twenty-one pounds), experienced this same doubt at the beginning of his course of instruction. "After so many years of suffering—on and off diets, up and down on the scale," he said, "I found it difficult to believe that all I had to do to slim down was to learn how to use more of the power of my mind. I tried everything else and failed, so I decided to go beyond my doubts and just do it ... every day. I'm glad I did, because I learned that most of those doubts and fears came from deep-down beliefs to the effect that I deserved to be 'punished' for eating so much over the previous years. So in order to lose that weight, I *had* to suffer ... by dieting.

"What ended my doubts was the new feeling that I deserved to be thin, regardless of past mistakes. Instead of punishing myself more, I started to treat myself with respect and kindness. I no longer thought in terms of 'how do I look' or 'what do people think of me.'

"Now, for the first time in my life, I feel great just being me."

It may be difficult for you, too, to accept the idea that you don't have to suffer to become a thin person. This thought arises from old programming and old beliefs about weight loss. But, by making the commitment to practice the Method daily, you will begin to experience its power to erase that faulty belief. When your self-image becomes "thin," there's no struggle staying that way.

Although the Method itself is easy to understand and to use, its simplicity requires effort. What takes the most consistent work on your part is the self-discipline it requires to set aside some time every day for practicing your new programming. Indeed, it takes discipline to ride a bike, give a speech, drive a car, or go to work. Ordinarily, you don't think of these things as needing discipline, but they do. Carrying out any decision requires discipline. In fact, discipline is part of your life-style.

Think about it...

Denise thought that she found a shortcut to rid herself of an excess ten pounds by using the Method only occasionally. Instead, it turned out to be a long detour. She worked for an ad agency and insisted her daily schedule was too crowded to allow time to practice the Method. She decided to practice once a week, hoping that her body would still benefit from the program.

"I now know this notion was ridiculous," she told me. "It was as silly as going to the doctor for medicine to cure an illness, leaving the bottle unopened on the shelf, and then complaining that the doctor wasn't making me well. Once I realized that I had been avoiding the discipline of daily practice, I started to do it every day. I began to look forward to it, because I was creating my thin self. It became one of the most enjoyable parts of my day. I like the idea of mental discipline. It makes so much sense, and I found that I was taking charge of my life."

Normally, when you hear the word *discipline*, you may think of something unpleasant or difficult. This isn't particularly true. Of course, discipline does require some effort on your part, but so does brushing your teeth. It, too, began as a discipline, and in time it became part of your daily routine.

Similarly, you must make the Method part of your daily routine. Rest assured the more you practice doing this, the less effort will be needed, until finally it becomes effortless.

Traveling a new road always has its bumpy passages. Think of anything you have mastered: passing your driving test (or trying to), learning how to play tennis (how many times were you embarrassed?), learning a new job skill, balancing your checkbook (if you're still working on this one, you're not alone!). You may have felt unsure about being able to do any of them at first, and you've probably forgotten your early, clumsy attempts. Until you persisted through the *entire learning process* and reduced it to a routine, you had not mastered the art.

It's the same with M.I.N.D. OVER WEIGHT®, with the singular characteristic of the process that some of its pitfalls are subtle. Therefore, you must be on the alert when it comes to dealing with your conscious mind, for until now your whole life-style has been regulated by it and you will meet resistance from it. After all, the familiar patterns that kept you overweight are being threatened by a new set of instructions you are programming it with. Your mind is not accustomed to *your* being in control of the way you think. It has gotten its way, whether it was "right" or "wrong."

It *is* a paradox. Here you are trying to improve your life by using wider areas of your mind, and yet your conscious reality resists the changes for the good. You may well ask why conscious reality is so perverse, since it consists of everything that you are aware of on a conscious level? It is the seat of your intellect—the knowledge and information you have acquired through study, education, reading. It is, in sum, your common sense, logic, rationale, and life experience— everything that makes up your conscious perception of the world. Surely, this consciousness must recognize how fat you are and how unhappy you are in this state?

Nonetheless, on your way to achieving your goal the conscious mind stubbornly creates roadblocks with a whole bag of deceitful tricks. Therefore, be on guard for mental excuses like "I'm too busy" (that's a good one), "I'm too tired," "I don't have time" (who's kidding whom?), "I don't feel like it" (this excuse covers it all!). The conscious mind is trying to prevent you from taking control of your life, resisting any change in its comfortable patterns—patterns that led to your weight problem in the past. Even though these habits may be hurtful to you, the outcome is predictable; therefore, the conscious mind is secure. Here you come, taking over with a new set of directions. You have become a threat to its dominion.

Whenever you hear that little voice cajoling, "You can't practice now," recognize it, be aware of it, and don't allow it to interfere with the free use of the Method. Remind yourself consciously that you are in charge of your life. Mental discipline of this kind involves selecting those thoughts that are good for you and using your conscious mind to redirect your subconscious thinking and beliefs.

For example, when you look in a mirror and see the bulge(s), don't say to yourself, "Wow, look at that fat! Boy, do I have a weight problem." Instead, look in the mirror, check out the bulge(s)—don't be afraid of them—and say to yourself, "Okay, they're there now, but I'm getting rid of them. I'm on my way to being a thin person." At that same moment, in your mind, see your image getting thinner and thinner. Enjoy it. It will start you off in the right direction for the rest of the day.

Studiously avoid the pitfall of making negative statements about yourself to others. When you're visiting a friend, and the subject turns to your current weight problem, as it often does with friends, what do you usually say to them about it? Do you find yourself repeating the same old phrases like "There's nothing I can do about it" or "I've tried everything and nothing works" or "I'll probably always have a weight problem." In effect, what you are doing is not only telling your friend, but *convincing yourself* you're a failure!

Clearly, negative statements are detrimental. They create unnecessary bumps on your road to success. Every time you think thoughts like these, or utter them, you are sending signals into your subconscious mind, where they'll be embedded—as faulty programming. Your efforts must be directed to positive, healthy, thin thoughts. Use good judgment and consider carefully what you say to yourself in order to design a new way of thinking about yourself. Thus, a positive consciousness is invited into your life which will activate newer, more positive feelings.

You'll begin to feel more confident even before the weight starts to melt away.

•

Remember Bob, the M.I.N.D.® student in Chapter 2 who believed he was doomed to be fat forever? He was a defeatist and believed he'd never be thin.

"What chance do I have," he rued. "My family keeps telling me I'll always be fat because *they* are."

Since he wasn't in a position to leave his family, Bob learned to use the Method to deal with the negative aspects of his home life. He realized that the major problem had been his *belief* in what his family kept telling him. What made matters worse was that Bob had been repeating these thoughts to himself, and consequently he had taken on *their* beliefs as *his* own. In spite of his family telling him that he could never hope to be thin, in spite of their belief that his weight problem was hereditary, Bob started to think slim, using the Method. When Bob began as a M.I.N.D. OVER WEIGHT® student, he was a 32-year-old businessman weighing over 320 pounds. At the end of one year, Bob weighed in at a comfortable 240 pounds, nicely distributed on his 6-feet, 3-inch frame. He achieved his success by not accepting negative statements as gospel truth, and by creating a positive consciousness. Today, Bob is in control and happy with his life. He still enjoys his family's culinary arts, but in moderation.

When you revise your conscious thinking like Bob did, you'll also find that you'll have a calmer, clearer mind. Your road to success will be smoother, with less anxiety and stress, because one of your greatest fears will have vanished—that is, your conscious fears about being overweight. To the degree you revise your conscious thinking and reprogram your subconscious beliefs about yourself, you set your conscious and subconscious mind in harmony, traveling a thin line in perfect balance.

•

Sometimes you may have to cope with a work environment that is onerous—the sort of place where the office becomes a mini-bakery at coffee-break time, offering a rich assortment of Danish, cakes, cookies, and doughnuts. This is a situation designed to sorely test the will power of any dieter.

Such was the case with Tracy.

Tracy was a nice young woman who worked in an office filled with other nice young women. She was having trouble getting rid of an extra ten pounds she didn't want, but no matter what she tried, she couldn't obtain her perfect shape. Another young woman in the office didn't suffer a weight problem; in fact, her measurements were ideal. She was a highly competitive person, and Tracy was her closest rival, so it gave her a lot of satisfaction to observe Tracy reaching for seconds at the coffee cart. One guess who bought the doughnuts? You're right. The doughnuts assured Tracy's erstwhile friend her own status as Number One in the office.

In working with the Method, Tracy became consciously aware of her own ability for self-control. Happily, today she's no longer compulsive about food. Not only did she lose those extra ten pounds, but no matter what sweet delights appear in the office, Tracy can have one or none, depending on how she feels. Anytime she gets an urge to eat too much, she says to herself, "Uh oh, I'm a thin person, and thin people don't eat like this!"

Of course, Tracy was not dealing only with her work environment. She was caught up in the competition. It can be very stimulating in some areas of living, but it's dangerous when you start to compete in weight-losing contests. In fact, quite often I hear remarks in seminars such as, "I'm annoyed at myself— I'm not losing as fast as other people" or "I was doing fine until I met my friend the other day. We started a weight-loss program together, and when I saw her, she had lost more than me. It makes me angry at myself and quite resentful toward her. I had to fast for a few days just to catch up!"

Have you ever found yourself doing this? If so, stop comparing yourself to others. You're only hurting yourself by playing this competitive game, and you end up focusing all your attention on someone else's success rather than on your own. Concentrate on yourself. To paraphrase an old adage, remember, you're marching to the sound of your own drummer. So if you find yourself in this kind of situation in the future, remind yourself that you're getting thin for you, *not* for someone else.

A great many people who try to lose weight convince themselves "I'm getting thin for my spouse" or "I'm getting thin for my mother" or "I'm getting thin for my fiancée" or "I'm getting thin for my children," and so on, and on. This is why they will *never* go the distance. They finish losers when they diet for someone else. Getting thin for someone else will create needless anxiety because of the constant comparisons to see if you measure up to what others are losing. Subtle remarks about how much you're eating, or "How much better you look when you are slim" are counterproductive. Ignore such observations. If you're trying to please everyone, you will certainly wind up pleasing no one, especially the one person who really counts—yourself!

Another situation you might run into while using the Method occurs when you're visiting relatives or friends who are not doing anything about their own overweight problem. They are liable to try all sorts of manipulations to get you to eat as much as they do. Watch out for these characters—the technique seldom fails, confirming that misery loves company. In the future, whenever you're with someone who tries to get you to overeat when you don't want to, remember that it's your choice now.

Have you thought about all those times you ate not because you were hungry, but because it was time for lunch, or time for dinner, or time for breakfast? There's no rule that says you *must* eat at a given time of day; this is especially true when you're not hungry. Examine your appetite before eating and you'll be amazed to discover that by doing this, you will eat no more than enough to satisfy that hunger.

As your eating habits change, people may ask you what diet you are on. They've noticed you getting thinner and not eating the way you used to eat. This is what happened to Hope.

"What do you mean, you're not on a diet? You can't lose weight without one!" everyone kept insisting to her. At first she found it difficult to explain that she was using her mind to lose weight. Someone remarked jokingly that Hope was "losing her mind, not losing weight," by thinking this way. But Hope stood her ground and could not be swayed. She let the doubters think what they wanted without trying to convince them otherwise. And the day came when it was obvious to Hope's friends that she *was* losing weight and she definitely was not eating diet foods. Curiosity took hold, and soon her friends were asking her serious questions.

In the past, Hope had been the object of whispered conversations, as there had been a whole lot of her to talk about. Now they speak of her success in maintaining a slim, delightful 140 pounds.

If friends ask *you* what you are doing to lose weight, tell them you're on a mental diet. Let the results speak for themselves.

Some of the other roadblocks that used to trigger your eating binges will no longer be a problem to you, like the tension and anxiety that demanded food for relief. Using the Method regularly will reduce many of the symptoms of stress; as for emotional crises with which you must cope, you'll be better equipped to deal with them through your expanded self-awareness—not through the refrigerator.

"I'm helpless," was Cathy's complaint when her friend brought her to see me. Cathy had a severe, rapid weight gain, adding 30 pounds to her original 120-pound body. In talking with her, I learned she was a 37-year-old housewife who recently had gone through the trauma of separation and divorce. It came unexpectedly and turned her life upside down, creating a lot of stress. She was anxious, confused, and quite emotional about the breakup. Moreover, relearning how to adjust to the singles scene was no easy task after having had a partner for more than fifteen years.

Now on shaky ground, unsure of herself, and unable to cope with a radical life-style change, she became a recluse—staying home most of the time, refusing invitations from her friends to "meet someone nice" at various parties. Nothing swayed her from this position. The more offers she got, the more she refused. To make matters worse, she was embarrassed about becoming overweight. Cathy had found a newer, safer "lover"—food!

She never had a weight problem before. It was all new to her. Her days and nights were so anxiety-ridden that she was having difficulty sleeping, and instead of going to bed, she sat up watching TV, snacking the entire time. When I introduced her to the Method, at first she wouldn't accept the idea that she could do anything to help herself. She already had failed on various diet regimens. Not only did she believe herself a failure because of her broken marriage, she was convinced she was a total failure who couldn't deal even with an increasingly troublesome weight problem. She told me that she decided to try the Method because she didn't have anything to lose—except the weight.

By using the Method, she was surprised to find that she was losing weight easily, at the rate of approximately eight pounds a month. Not only that, she was no longer spending every spare moment *thinking* about food. Her healthy self-image was reemerging, stronger than ever. She took the plunge into her new life-style and soon discovered that she could handle it; she enjoyed the adventure of meeting new people and going to new places. She was back in the stream of life again—back on the thin road.

It's been over a year since I saw Cathy, and she called me recently to tell me that she's more confident than ever. She has a full-time job she loves, she has maintained her slim figure of 120 pounds, and she has no fear of feeling helpless again.

Remember the trigger mechanisms listed in the multiple-choice test in Chapter 2? These "binge buttons" may have caused an automatic response in you because of some faulty programming. Maria had one devastating binge button—anger. She was angry much of the time at many people, and it became a serious problem. When she experienced anger, she ran for food. If she wasn't angry at someone else, she became angry at herself for one reason or another.

It proved enlightening for her to discover that she wasn't becoming angry as often since using the Method. Her mental mini-vacation each day was paying off. She became clearer and more aware of why she was responding to anger by feeding herself. She came to recognize that she was abusing herself by overeating because she felt ashamed at her anger; so to avoid greater emotional explosion, she soothed her feelings with the balm of food.

Currently, Maria is dealing more effectively with her anger, making it smaller all the time, and her body is responding similarly.

A major roadblock that causes problems is the guilt of overeating. Guilt is one of the most dangerous of the binge buttons: First you overeat, then you feel guilty, then you overeat to ease the pain of *that* guilt. Therefore, it is important to realize that guilt is a manufactured product, produced in your mind, and you can interrupt that assembly-line process. If you find that you are overeating, don't spend time feeling guilty, but redirect your thoughts toward the reasons behind the guilt/overeating cycle. Avoid blaming yourself, and revise your thoughts and feelings about yourself so that they are benign and self-accepting. The same is true with your fears about gaining weight because of a rare overeating incident. Don't worry. You'll probably find that for a few days afterward you won't have too great an appetite. This is your mind's natural way of compensating for the overindulgence.

By working regularly with the Method, you are deactivating those old binge buttons. Remember Lisa, who felt anger at her mother and guilt at herself for overeating? In her case, there were two triggers that kept her on a regular course of failure. However, working with the Method helped her stop "swallowing her anger" at her mother. Instead, she started communicating her feelings to her mother until they reached a new understanding of their relationship. Soon the overeating and induced vomiting ceased, and Lisa has continued to maintain her weight loss of 30 pounds for three years.

Now your journey begins, and it's time for you to take your place in the thin parade. It's where you really belong. You deserve it. Walk the thin line with confidence ... walk with new awareness of yourself.

Chapter 7

STAY THIN FOREVER... NATURALLY

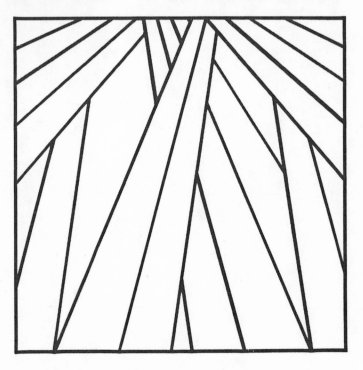

What your mind wills, will be. You control your mind through your thoughts and beliefs. Choose to *think* and *believe* slim. By doing the Method regularly, you summon an inner ability to remain slim for the rest of your life. The manifestation of the dream of being thin forever comes when you have accepted the thin reality that can exist in your mind. Isn't it marvelous to discover that what you have been looking for has been with you all along? This power is not unusual or extraordinary—it is a natural ability everyone possesses: the ability of mind to control body.

Today there is enormous interest in the potential of the human mind. Open your favorite magazine or newspaper, turn on your TV, and you are exposed to new findings concerning the mind's powers. Yet for aeons, sages have been telling us, in effect, that there is more to us than meets the eye. They foretold the untapped potential of the human mind that we are only now beginning to comprehend.

Modern scientists in their laboratories are substantiating what heretofore was simply theory and conjecture. In fact, modern medical science is doing more varieties of research into the mind-body relationship, and a new branch of medicine has emerged in recent decades devoted to the study of psychosomatic illness. (The word *psychosomatic* itself is derived from *psyche*, which means mind or spirit, and *soma*, which means body.) Consequently, many ailments are being recognized as having their origins *in the mind*. All of these new findings are based on the attainment of a higher level of consciousness, reaching beyond the recognized limitations of the conscious mind.

Higher consciousness or any altered condition of consciousness is a state of mind that is different from ordinary, waking consciousness. One of the clearest demonstrations of mind over matter is exhibited by the popular art of karate. Have you ever watched average people breaking planks of wood or smashing cinder blocks with one chop of the hand? Next time you do, notice the concentration on the face of the individual as he or she prepares to accomplish such a feat. Certainly this person is not thinking, "I'm going to hurt my hand when I strike this." On the contrary, the attention is totally focused on the end *result*. There is no thought of pain or damage to the hand. They have psyched themselves into a higher state of consciousness, and the consciousness is fully directed toward *success*; so the arm and hand are, seemingly, transformed into steel.

You have the same power to apply similarly toward the object of becoming and remaining slim. Keep *your* attention fully focused on your desired goal. Utilize the higher level of consciousness produced by practicing the Method, and you will direct your mind to successfully control your body weight.

There are many different ways to raise the consciousness. I chose to use the meditative approach as the consciousness raiser for M.I.N.D. OVER WEIGHT®. I preferred meditation because we could do it ourselves, do it alone, do it anywhere, and do it simply. The word meditation has its root in the Latin verb *meditari*, which simply means to contemplate, to ponder, to keep the mind or attention fixed upon (some object). It has been used successfully over the centuries to discipline the mind and expand its powers. The benefits of practicing meditation include the development of a calm self-control and an expanded self-awareness.

Meditation is not a new concept; in fact, it is

thousands of years old, well-known to most Eastern cultures. We found that it could be adapted to fill the needs of Western society—of people living in a hectic world with all its stress and anxiety.

Having learned this ancient art, we found that by actively utilizing the relaxed state of the body and alertness of the mind—the meditative space—we could see things more clearly, and understand better how our minds worked. From this platform we discovered we could direct the power of our minds toward a chosen result and accomplish a selected goal in an active, effective way. We incorporated into the Method the techniques of visualization to create a new, healthy self-image, and to embed this mental picture firmly in the subconscious mind.

Meditation itself is a tension reliever having cumulative effects. Not only do you feel calmer and clearer during the practice period, but that feeling continues throughout the day. You'll feel physically more relaxed and mentally more alert; and as you pass through the novice stage to become more proficient (after a week or two of regular practice), you'll notice that you're less tense.

You'll also find that the meditative aspect of the Method will produce the space in your mind needed to get in touch with your subconscious beliefs. You'll be pleased at how rewarding it is to change faulty beliefs and old programmings. Thus your self-image will change, keeping step with newer, healthier beliefs. An improved self-image will bring many welcome changes to your life-style as you begin to experience a newfound sense of self-respect. You'll find yourself walking tall, with a greater sense of ease and confidence than ever before.

You'll be more aware of your thinking processes,

and you'll begin to understand *how* your mind works. Instead of automatically *reacting* to situations that caused you to overeat in the past, you'll now be able to *act* wisely. You will be in control of your body, and *aware* of the way you function. Those binge buttons will become inoperative.

Letting go of past mistakes is possible after you've examined them at a higher level of consciousness. After you have *seen* them clearly in your mind, *recognized* them as having been detrimental, and *understood* how these misconceptions held you back from a thin life, only then will you be able to release them. Once they are gone, they won't be able to hurt you anymore. Start to spend some time looking at your good points: qualities in yourself that you admire, your successful achievements. Accentuate your positive characteristics. An expanded self-awareness provides the opportunity for you to get to know yourself better. The more you *look* at your good points, the more you'll *like* yourself. You'll stop judging yourself so harshly. Make a habit of checking out your good points regularly. And enjoy feeling *good* about yourself.

By forming your mental blueprint every day, you will actualize the image. Remember, imagination is the essence of creation—the real power behind your thoughts and beliefs. The use of imagination is more potent when you are in a state of higher consciousness. As you visualize yourself as the perfect, thin you, and experience those positive, powerful emotions, you are sending strong pictures into your subconscious mind.

By not dieting you will get out of the overweight frame of mind and move away from that consciousness which was preoccupied with food. Fear of food reduces the concentration of power you are directing toward your goal. Therefore, focus your attention on the positive end result, and think about food in terms of its nutritional value to the health of your body without sacrificing the pleasurable aspects of eating. If you are not certain of a good nutritional eating program, consult your physician, who can recommend one that is best for your health.

Losing weight without a diet is a very natural process. Now your *mind* will direct you to eat the way you need to in order to be a thin person. Your appetite will change accordingly. Follow the process—it *will* happen for you.

All the ingredients for a permanently thin life are now at your disposal. You have an opportunity to work on yourself, by yourself, and for yourself *at your own pace.* The M.I.N.D. OVER WEIGHT® method will work for you, so pursue it with enthusiasm and confidence.

You won't have to rely on elements outside yourself to achieve success. Every benefit that you enjoy by using the Method will happen as a result of your own efforts. Opening your mind in this way is like waking from a deep sleep. You will start to see things differently. Life will become much clearer because you will play a more active role in determining how things will go for you.

This moment is the beginning of the rest of your life. Why not make a commitment to yourself to enjoy it fully? This is *your* life. Get thin for *yourself.* Give *yourself* this gift, and those around you will also benefit.

You constitute your entire world; it is composed

of your feelings, your emotions, your perceptions of life and its realities and illusions. Stop for a moment to consider how important you really are. Consider the fact that there is only one of you, that you are unique, that there's not another person like you anywhere in the world. You are an original. That's why you're so special.

There will come a time when you will no longer *need* to formally practice the Method. Once the belief in the thin you has become a reality, you'll maintain your desired weight by effortlessly maintaining the desired thoughts. In time, thinking and believing slim will become *knowing*. You'll develop a certainty about the permanence of your thin life, a knowledge that goes beyond thought or aspiration. And when you *know*, nothing can take you away from it, ever!

> *"What lies behind us and what lies before us are but tiny matters compared to what lies within us."*
>
> Ralph Waldo Emerson

Think about it...